Healing Hearts

Paula Schneider, RN, MPH
Editor

Judy, may you find the spirit of healing in this book and pass it on.

Paula Schneider
8/1/99

Vista Publishing, Inc.

Copyright © 1999 by Paula Schneider

Edited by Paula Schneider, RN, MPH

Cover Design by Thomas Taylor of Thomcatt Graphics

Vista Publishing, Inc.
422 Morris Avenue, Suite One
Long Branch, NJ 07740
(732) 229-6500

This publication is designed for the reading pleasure of the general public. In order to ensure confidentiality, the names of all patients and physicians have been changed or omitted. In some cases, the names of clinics, hospitals, and other institutions have been altered as well. Nurses who wish to remain anonymous have been granted their wish, and their biographies are not included. The subjects of the story, "Viola's Choice," specifically requested the names remain intact in memory of Viola, and that request was honored.

Printed and bound in the United States of America

First Edition

ISBN: 1-880254-61-1
Library of Congress Catalog Card Number: 99-71045

U.S.A. Price: $16.95
Canada Price: $21.95

Acknowledgments

I would like to express my gratitude to my husband, Larry, for being my best friend, mentor, and biggest supporter throughout the last 18 months. He has given me daily encouragement, and would not allow me to give up in my darkest hours. He has always seen the highest and best in me and continually reminds who I am and that I have a unique gift to give to the world.

Our dear friends and playmates, Ray and Cindy Dix, have redefined the meaning of friendship for me. We have spent countless hours together, visualizing this book nurturing millions of people throughout the world, as it becomes the success we know it is destined to be.

Much gratitude goes to my Powerful Women's MasterMind partners: Clare Rice, my mentor and friend; Penny Hunt, who always sees the best in everyone; Dr. Elisabeth Stein, a radiant being who always gives me words of positive encouragement; and Linda Roberts, a smiling friend who supports unconditionally.

And last but not least, I am overwhelmed to find the right words of gratitude for the beautiful nurses who have made this book possible. Without them, there would be no book! Many of them have taken the best their hearts have to offer, formed it into special words of love and giving, and offered it to the readers of this book. Their stories have touched and enriched me, brightened my day, turned my smiles into tears of joy and thanksgiving, and have lifted me to a new and special place that feeds my soul.

My wish is that these stories will move you the same way.

Dedication

With my heart full of gratitude for the gifts given to me as a result of preparing this book, I dedicate these stories to the loving spirit that flows throughout the universe. Thank you for reminding us, through these shared experiences, that caring creates communication, and at that point of unity true healing emerges.

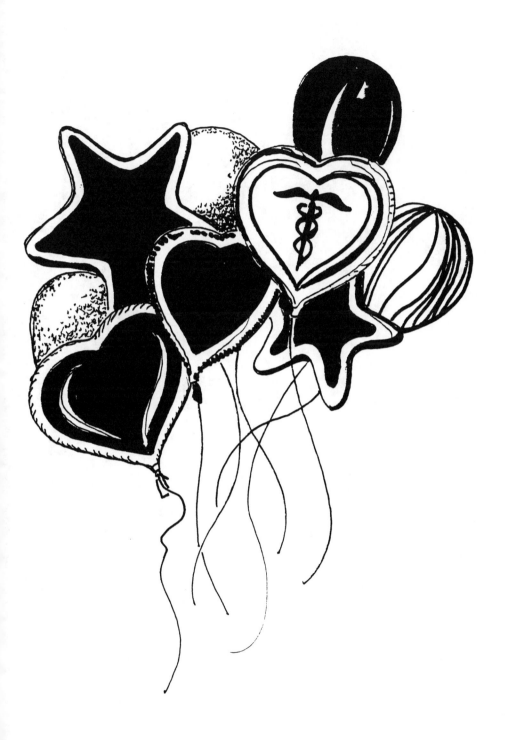

Table of Contents

Introduction

1. ***The Wind That Lifts Us Up***   ***1-39***
      It Looks Like Rain Today   2
      Mimi   4
      Will I Be Able to Walk in Heaven?   6
      Shalom, Jennie   8
      A Measure of Time   10
      It's All Perspective   13
      The Edge of the Bed   16
      A Hospice Death   19
      My Little Greek Friend   21
      The Blizzard and The Flood   22
      The Love of God   23
      Shades of White   25
      Whose Call Is It?   29
      Naked Cora   31
      Thank You, Aunt Tommie   34
      Easing Her Pain   36
      Viola's Choice   37

2. ***Breaking the Illusion***   ***40-66***
      Angel in the Black Robe   41
      Visiting Hours   42
      Sam and Eva   45
      Anxious to Leave   49
      Unfinished Business   51
      It's Time to Release Him   52
      Nina's Angel   54
      This Death   56
      The Light   58
      Waiting for Her Son   60
      A Final Message of Love and Hope   61
      My Angel Has Come Back   63
      Divine Intervention   64
      Immune Suppressed Unit 1330   65

Table of Contents

3. **The Essence of Care Giving: Serving With Love**   **67-100**
    Just to Be There   68
    The Haitian Baby   69
    Nursing is Unique   71
    The Caring Lesson   73
    Hope   75
    A Twist of Fate   77
    Nursing: My Commitment and Reward   79
    I Teach   81
    My Job, My Calling   82
    Diary of a New Nurse   84
    I Understand   86
    Our Team Leaders, the Elderly   88
    Angels Away at Camp   89
    A Chance to Touch   90
    Circle of Life   92
    The Lightning Ridge Experience   96
    We'll Meet Again Some Day   98
    Creative Solutions   100

4. **Humor Lightens the Load**   **101-120**
    The Sundowner   102
    The Impersonator   104
    Hmm, Hmm Good   105
    Ms. Clara's Peanut Butter Sandwiches   106
    Nurse Knows Best   108
    The Bath   109
    No More Cruises for Mavis!   110
    The Nose Knows   112
    Giggles from the Psychiatric Unit   113
    Junior 007 and The Young Lady in White   115
    A Foot Stomping Time   117
    The Payoff   119
    What Time Is It?   120

Table of Contents

5. *Medical Stretches*   *121-135*
      Our Miracle Lady   122
      Mr. Fuller   123
      Just Another Day at School   125
      I Will Lead the Blind   127
      The Christmas Miracle   130
      She Wasn't Ready Yet!   132
      Just Lupus   133

Biographies   *136-144*

About the Editor   *145*

Introduction

Healing From the Heart is an anthology of inspirational stories written by nurses about events and special patients in our professional lives. Contributors live in Australia, Singapore, Canada, England, and the United States. We work in virtually all areas of nursing, and our ages range from new nurse to mature nurse. This captivating collection of true stories uplifts the spirits and reminds us what healing, caring, and giving are all about.

Nurses have been a constant in the healing arts. Historically, nurses were midwives and were called upon to provide herbal remedies for conditions ranging from stomach distress to broken bones to normal pregnancy and delivery. We provided comfort in times of need and held hands when all hope of recovery had vanished. We medicated with teas, soups, salves, potions, poultices, and love. Some were even called witches because our healing methods were misunderstood and feared.

Today's nurse works in a high technology, sometimes impersonal, world of machines, intravenous and tube feedings, and electrical devices that monitor every aspect of the human body's activities. We are challenged every day to maintain high levels of technical skills and abilities while finding the time to hold a hand or soothe a worried brow. In the current managed care atmosphere of down-sizing, right-sizing, and fiscal cutbacks which directly impact patient care, nurses today find ourselves in very difficult situations where we must decide which type of care is more important, because we no longer have sufficient time or staffing to do both.

This book is dedicated to all nurses, past, present, and future. We have served well, and if we have touched just one life and made it easier to survive a crisis, then we have achieved our mission.

I hope you will be inspired, touched, and uplifted by the genuine, from-the-heart stories you will read in **Healing From the Heart**. They are for *YOU*.

Paula Schneider, RN, MPH

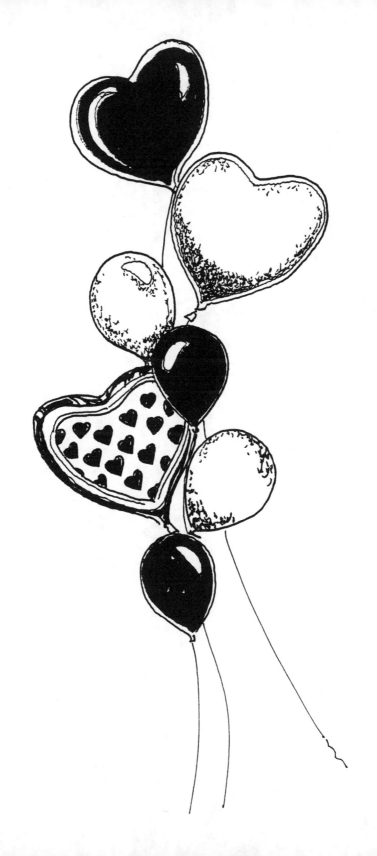

1

The Wind That Lifts Us Up

Every day, nurses have experiences that validate who we are and what we do. Now, we share with you some of these memories. We have held hands, cried, rejoiced, sat with dying patients as they took their last breath, and told family members that their beloved would not be returning. We consider these special, intimate, and sometimes holy times, and we are honored to be present for them. Read now what nurses wish to share about these priceless moments shared with patients, and be renewed.

It Looks Like Rain Today

Tee Angel

An assault on the senses—that's all I could think about after being in the nursing home for 15 minutes. My vision of a "nursing home" is lots of caring and nurturing. This was much more like a nightmare gone very wrong. How can anyone find solace here? It felt desolate to be among so many disjointed fragments of life. I had to stop a moment to catch my own senses in order to understand their world as it is, not how I envision it to be. These are the sounds that surround my patients. I cannot be a part of their world without understanding that. I must not filter out the cries that line the halls like psychedelic paper.

I go to my first patient of the day. She lies sleeping in her bed while another woman in a wheelchair collects wire hangers from a worn and tired dresser. She wheels around to confront me using one toe of her right foot. She moved yesterday—these hangers are hers. She is waiting for her husband, gone many years ago. She speeds off with all the might that one toe can muster. I turn back to my patient, resting peacefully in her bed. I stroke her cheek, she looks up at me and smiles a warm and loving smile, filled with so much hope that my heart breaks. Then she asks, "What have I done wrong?" I hold her face in my hands, and visit with her until she nods off to sleep.

The sisters are next, Millie and Elle. They are ending their lives as they began it—in a room shared only as sisters can share, each connected to the other in the way they alone understand. Millie is experiencing cancer and will soon die, yet she is full of life and joy. Elle carries her sister's pain to the point that she can barely move. We sit looking out the windows, watching the gardeners clearing away the freshly cut debris from the grounds. Clearing away the dead and dying. When asked about her view of health, Millie says, "Today is like a wind. I have lived and conquered." Her words are a source of strength for me. I know that she means she is at peace with dying.

2

Then, as quickly as she is present in the moment, she is gone. Looking out onto the bright blue of the sky, she says, "It looks like rain today." And, I knew in that moment, there was a mist I could not see pressing against the window, placing a haze on her view of the day. It passes the pane and settles into Millie's soul. No thunder or lightning in a violent rush, but a slow creeping bog of cool, wet soil caressing her gently within its grasp. Time, not cancer, has called for Millie. She will pass, not with pain, but with the lightness of the mist in a gentle rain.

I leave Millie and Elle, realizing that the sounds that assaulted me are not important. What is important is the acknowledgement of having lived life well. The collective voice pleading for recognition of their value and worth—a voice filled with dignity. They have done nothing wrong...

Mimi

Susan Kirkland

Mimi McLaughlin arrived in the recovery room at 3:10 AM, still under anesthesia. I began baseline vital signs, positioned her oxygen mask, and examined her casted left arm. She stabilized quickly, and after the surgeon's report and a second visit from the anesthesiologist, Mimi and I were alone.

When I began the fourth set of vital signs, her eyes popped open, and she surprised me with a smile. "Hello." Her eyes were bright blue and twinkling and very youthful for her 88 years. "I thought I saw an angel, but it's you."

"No wings or halos, Mimi. Just your recovery room nurse."

"Didn't make it to heaven this time, did I?"

"Not your time yet. Guess you'll just have to stay here with us mortals for a while longer."

"Oh, I don't mind. Not really. My mission is still not complete, I suppose."

"Mission?" I asked. "What kind of mission?"

"My children. Teaching. Been teaching for many years. Children are my life." What a charming, funny, and intelligent lady! She told me how she came to our "grand" country as a young girl from Aberdeen, Scotland. There was still a hint of a Scottish brogue. She had no complaints of pain, and she simply ignored the heavy cast placed on her small arm after she took a nasty fall at home.

"I've lived in a small house near Adams School for many years. After I retired, my home became a safety stop for the children who walked to and from school. If they get caught in the rain or need assistance, my house is a haven for them."

"I drive by Adams School on my route to work. I believe I've seen you in the window. A white Cape Cod style with blue shutters?"

"That's me," she said proudly. "I keep an eye on the little ones.

4

When you go by, Sara, just tap your car horn. I'll wave to you."

And so began a routine that lasted for several years. Mimi was always there, sitting near the window. She smiled and waved as I drove by. A shawl of red plaid covered her shoulders, and with her white hair positioned in a little bun, she was a sweet picture.

I had been away on vacation for several weeks, and returning to work, I noticed that Mimi's house stood empty. The following day, I stopped to speak with her neighbor.

"She's gone to live with her son. He has begged her for years, but she loved the children here. She was principal of Adams School for 20 years, and taught there for 30. Mimi was a wonderful neighbor and loved by everyone."

"Where is she living?" I asked, thinking I would write just to say I missed her.

The woman looked at me with a puzzled frown. "With her son, his wife, and her grandchildren, of course—in the Governor's mansion."

Will I Be Able to Walk in Heaven?

Chris Shirey

J.G., Hispanic, 10 years old, AIDS, tumor of the spinal cord probably related to HIV infection, due for surgery to remove the tumor, possibility of permanent paralysis after surgery. My little patient, my young friend of four years, has just been told that he might be paralyzed or may die as a result of the surgery, and he is frightened. His mother, also infected with HIV, is either unwilling or unable to discuss his disease with her son. Not able to offer emotional support, J.G.'s mother often tells him, "Relax," "Be brave," or "Have hope." J.G.'s father is an alcoholic, and is physically and emotionally removed from the family. To add to this sad scenario, J.G. has a three-year-old brother who is severely retarded. J.G. takes an active role in his brother's life, in caring for him and encouraging him to perform daily activities.

Today is the day before surgery, and I visit with J.G. in his private hospital room. As I arrive, I run into his mother who tells me in Spanish that she is going home to take care of the three-year-old. J.G. appears anxious that his mother is leaving, and is crying and begging her not to leave. She gives him her stock reply, "Relax. Be brave," and tears out the door. I hasten to J.G.'s bedside, and we get down to business.

"Please don't leave, Chris. I don't want to be alone," he pleads.

"I'm here with you. I won't leave," I reassure.

"I'm scared."

I ask, "What are you scared of?"

"They are going to cut me tomorrow and they told me I might be paralyzed."

"That's scary," I sympathetically reply.

"The doctor said I might die," J.G. whispered as his eyes pierced the depths of my soul. "If they paralyze my legs, do you think I'll be able to walk in heaven?"

Knots form in my throat as I struggle to answer. The words finally

6

come, "I don't know. But I think heaven is supposed to be a place where everything is perfect and you feel no pain, so I think you would be able to walk. Is that what you are scared of the most?"

"No. I want to know who will take care of my little brother when I'm gone." This precious little angel is facing major surgery tomorrow, and he's more concerned about his little brother than himself. Oh, that we could all be this selfless! Then, we go on to talk about what heaven and death are like, and about our feelings and fears. J.G., justifiably, has plenty of fears today.

He wants to see his little brother, so I arrange a visit for tonight. The neurosurgeon drops by and reassures J.G. that the surgery risks are one on a scale of one to 10, offering hope to my frightened patient, and I hold his hand as he drifts off to sleep. I am prepared to spend the night at J.G.'s bedside if his parents don't return.

J.G. is facing an overwhelming list of burdens and fears at this moment, problems that most of us will never have to face in this lifetime. His mother, working with her own beliefs and probable denial, is unable to offer support. He is, truly, alone on this formidable journey through life.

While caring for J.G., I have been given the opportunity to face some of my own fears. "Will he die during surgery (He is my friend!)?" "Will he be paralyzed?" "Can I deal with his possible death?" "Why would God let little children suffer?" "Can I help J.G.? If so, how?"

I believe I alleviated a small portion of J.G.'s anxiety just by listening to his concerns and holding his hand. When he asked me if he would be able to walk in heaven, I was filled with sadness, knowing he'd been thinking about this for some time. Wishing for concrete facts to give him, I instead answered from my heart when I reassured him that it is my personal belief that heaven is a wonderful place where there is no suffering. I was filled with awe that even though he is terminally ill, J.G. is still so concerned about his younger brother. Truly, I am privileged to have this little angel touch my life!

P.S. J.G. survived the surgery, without paralysis, and today runs and plays with his little brother.

Shalom, Jennie

Naomi Follis

The first time I saw Jennie she was being escorted down the long hallway of the nursing home in her wheelchair, accompanied by her son and daughter-in-law. Her blonde-tinged wig was arranged neatly on her head and a touch of blush was on her pale cheeks. The soft blue eyes glistened as she was shown the room that would be her last earthly home.

Jennie was accustomed to the finest that life had to offer. Born a Jewish immigrant in Russia, she married the handsome and prosperous Sam, in her youth. His lucrative chain of jewelry stores reached from New York to Oklahoma. With the senior Sam now deceased, the business rested in the capable hands of their only child, Sam Junior.

The adjustment to the nursing home went much smoother than was anticipated and Jennie was soon acclimated to the mundane routine. Her charming stories of her lovely home always ended with her soulful declaration, "That was then, this is now-- things change."

The years crept by; age took its toll on Jennie, extracting its due, for the time allotted on earth. She no longer wore the wig or the huge, round designer glasses that dwarfed her elfin face.

Her hearing bad, she yelled out her wishes as if we were the ones hard of hearing. Often she would revert to her native Russian or Yiddish when speaking. Her son, Sam, constantly reminded her, "English, Mom, English."

Many times, as she sat in her wheelchair, she looked up to the ceiling and talked to God, asking in her thick accent, "God, do you hear me? God, are you home?"

One day, as she sat alone, asking the same questions, a mischievous employee passed by and yelled back, "Yeah!" Jennie didn't take her eyes off the ceiling but raised her hands to gesture upward and in her finest Yiddish accent said, "So what? You just got in?"

Shortly after her 95th birthday, we began to notice that Jennie was starting to lose weight. Her tiny body was becoming more and more frail. The food on her supper tray disappeared for the most part, so it remained a mystery as to the cause of the weight loss. One evening, out of the corner of my eye, I noticed Jennie stealthily storing the food in her napkin. I watched as she wheeled herself down the hallway from the dining room and deposited bits of food wherever she thought no one would find them. In spite of the dietary supplements we gave her, it became apparent that Jennie would soon leave us.

Her vital signs began to diminish as I sat by her side, and held her hand. The long, graceful fingers were cold, and signs of strain showed on her tired face.

Her breathing was shallower now, and I leaned close to her ear and said, "It's okay, Jennie, you can rest now. Go for the light. I promise you, God is home."

An almost undetectable smile tugged at the corners of her mouth and an angelic look of peace crossing her pale face and her breathing ceased.

"Shalom, Jennie, Shalom."

A Measure of Time

Tee Angel

Clouds of blue sky merging in the distance;

Two spirits in unison;

Streams locked in by land surround their refuge;

Nature's carpet, lush and vibrant, sends the smell of rich dark earth to
lungs of long ago;

Breezes blowing strength and hope – caressing the windows as
they brush

Past – touching hair which flows in loving disarray;

Breasts which nurture, filled with life, pools of warmth and light –
breasts of passion

Creating the walls of love to hold them tight;

Transcendence to a greater good;

Bastions of truth and beauty;

Subtle shifts to many realms where time IS
measured...

By a watch that has no hands.

As I cross the threshold at my first home visit of the day, I move between dimensions. The house becomes a home, and these people become persons. I feel the shift within myself, a gentle awakening flowing through my inner self which opens my nursing practice to all the possibilities this home has to offer. I take a moment to look around the room. This is important in gaining insight into their lives, hopes, and dreams. It is uncomfortable at first—it feels like an invasion into their private world. The invasion is without intent to do harm, so I let the feeling pass by acknowledging its relevance, or lack thereof, to this situation. I look past the obvious—the furniture, carpet, and wallpaper—to the heart of the home. The love within a home is always stored in a unique way or place. Here, I have found it on the walls.

There are women everywhere. Paintings, drawings, sketches—all with the shapes and forms of women. Nudes contrast with robes of many colors. Black and white against passionate reds. Breasts filled with life, love, and hope. The love of this home is nurturing.

Then I meet them, and they are in love. The years have made them one in spirit. How can one part of a united spirit pass on without the other? The calls for nursing cried out from the very walls. Her call asks, "Can we go on as one when he is no longer here in body?" She does not think of going with him on this journey, but of how she can keep him here, in spirit, for hers. She continues to hem his pants, arrange his clothes, and plan his meals. She asks questions as a way to continue to provide his care. She strives to keep her promise that she will be there with him, in their home, when he passes on.

His calls are delicate, yet strong. He wants to be with her, for she is his life. "Honey" never tastes so sweet or smells so good as it does when he speaks to her. He calls to be seen as her lover, friend, husband, mate, provider, caretaker, caregiver. Whole in this moment. He wants to die at home surrounded by the nurturing of all the women on the walls, the women who make up the many sides of her, his wife.

As I enter this home, the wind pouring through the windows carries hope. It is not hope in the sense that he will not die, or that they will spend many more years together. But, it is hope for the present, hope for living out these precious minutes to the fullest; open to the possibilities that transcend time.

Holding his hand, I look down, wanting to see his hand in mine. I watch our clasped fingers and feel the connection between our common human spirit within the world we have just created. The winds blow through my hair that brushes against my cheek, and I know we have shifted to an even higher place. I look at the watch on his wrist and realize that time has no meaning here—it is only a symbol—for the hands lie in disarray beyond the crystal, broken from the face where time used to be.

It's All Perspective

Paula Schneider

As I turned my little maroon Toyota X-Cab pickup onto the bumpy and dusty country lane, I wondered what gifts my next patient would give me. You see, I believe all my patients are my teachers if I will but stay awake and listen. It's funny to think that we believe we are there just to perform some technical task or another, when the secret is, they come into our world to offer us a lesson.

"So," I contemplated as I continued down the road, "my challenge is to discover what this patient has to tell me." I would soon find out. After a seemingly endless ride from the paved county road into a country subdivision of mobile and modular homes, I pulled into his yard. As I approached the older model mobile home, I quickly noticed shreds of insulation hanging down from the entire bottom of the home. I made a mental note to ask about this later on (turns out the dogs had shredded it a few months back and it hadn't been repaired yet).

Mr. O'Malley was an elderly gentleman, legally blind, with an indwelling catheter draining urine directly from his bladder through his abdomen into a collection bag. He had a large lesion on his leg that had not responded to periodic office visits to his doctor 20 miles away. Mrs. O'Malley was unable to help care for her husband, as she had her own emotional health problems to keep her occupied. So, there they were 20 miles out in the middle of nowhere, attempting to live comfortably while resisting going to an assisted living facility for as long as they could. Their daughter and her husband lived a short distance away, and they did what they could to help their parents. It was definitely an interesting situation!

My orders were to soak Mr. O'Malley's leg for 20 minutes in an Epsom salts solution, dry the leg and lesion, apply Silvadene crème, and wrap the leg with gauze. This was to be done daily until the leg began to heal. Thus began my first challenge: finding a pail deep enough to cover the lesion, which was fairly high on his shin. Mrs. O'Malley brought me a tall kitchen trash can, plastic, dirty, and smelly with old food residue. I had to wash it well with soap and water before I could use it.

Then came the challenge of the soak. The mobile home was not air conditioned, even though it was almost 100 degrees that day. Electing to sit out on the tin-roofed, screened porch on aluminum chairs with worn and broken webbing, Mr. O'Malley and I talked as he soaked. He cheerfully recounted episodes from his past, and kept us both entertained for 20 minutes. Our talk was interrupted frequently by the barnyard cats who quickly realized the owners were busy and took advantage of this opportunity to dart through holes in the screen into the house in hopes of finding a scrap of food. Mr. O'Malley attempted to shoo them out, to no avail. The time passed quickly, even though my uniform was wet with perspiration as we baked in the Florida sun.

After the dressing change was completed, I went inside the trailer to wash my hands and discard used supplies. The odor of old food was overpowering as I approached the kitchen area. As I passed through the living area, I noticed the carpet was stained with what was most likely spilled urine. That odor and the stale food odor combined to create a most unpleasant smell. I looked around for Mrs. O'Malley and found her in bed in a room that had only plywood flooring—no carpet or rugs. The room was a mess, much like the rest of the house. I saw a few live roaches as I continued through the hallway on the way to a lavatory. Needless to say, this was not a good living situation at all, and I made mental notes that I intended to share with my home health agency supervisor when I got back to the office, 40 miles away.

It turned out that Mr. O'Malley had been a patient of the agency for many months. Originally, we saw him for catheter changes only, and we provided a home health aide who helped him with a shower three times a week. Everyone in the office, including social workers, knew of the unfavorable living conditions, but after much research into his case, the decision was made that this was not a case of elder abuse. The daughter was clearly doing all she could within her means to ensure her parents' medical and everyday needs were met. Even though perhaps not meeting some of our personal standards, the O'Malley's were clothed, fed, clean, and receiving proper medical care.

I visited Mr. O'Malley daily for over a month, during which time I grew to have a deep admiration and respect for him. This was a gentleman who never once complained about his lot in life, even though it

14

was clear to me he was financially impoverished. He often met me at the door dressed only in boxer shorts, and when he did wear shorts or long pants, they were filled with holes and were ill-fitting. He made it clear to me that he felt very lucky. Happily married, he enjoyed living in the peace and quiet of the country and felt he had everything he needed to be happy. He always greeted me with a big, toothless smile, and never failed to thank me for coming to visit. On one occasion, my husband accompanied me on a late afternoon visit, and after that, Mr. O'Malley always asked about him. He was a person who could step outside his surroundings to think about other people.

So, Mr. O'Malley became my teacher. He helped me understand that worldly possessions aren't always necessary for happiness—that true joy comes from **within**. Fully accepting the fact that he would always need a catheter for urinary drainage, he never once complained to me about that burden. In fact, I don't remember him complaining about anything (even though it took over three months to get his leg healed)!

I was the student here. I watched, I listened, and I learned. That, to me, is what makes nursing one of the richest professions that one can go into. Few other vocations offer, on a daily basis, the opportunity to interact with people on such a deep and meaningful level. What a wonderful gift and growth opportunity!

The Edge of the Bed

Mary Arnold

Finally! The summer semester of 1978 was here. I had ended my first year of nursing school and was looking forward to my obstetrical rotation. After having spent the last semester in psychiatric facilities, shelters, and funeral homes, I was ready for smiles.

My instructor was Frances Brown, a mother hen of the instruction contingency. She was heavy set, matronly, silver-haired, and soft spoken with kind eyes and gentle hands. We all gravitated toward her, hence the mother hen analogy. Wherever she went, there were students milling around her like baby chicks. EVERYTHING she said was significant!

My patient had delivered a premature baby in the middle of the night, and the baby had been rushed to a larger hospital hundreds of miles away for specialized care. My tearful patient was in desperate need of a bath, so I set to work in the best student nurse form—scrubbing, combing, lotioning, and repositioning. She never said a word, only cried. I tried to coax her into talking about her experience, because as all students knew, we had to go at the end of the day to a post-clinical conference to share our pearls of wisdom with our fellow students. So, I tried a variety of topics, but my patient only wanted to cry. There she was with a clean bed, freshly scrubbed and clothed, and she was still crying...I had to DO something...but what should I DO? I had DONE everything I knew how to DO...I stood there, and then it hit me...Mother Hen! I pulled up my patient's side rail (good student nurses always put up the rails), and ran to find Mrs. Brown.

Just the sight of her was enough to cause me to burst into tears of despair. I had not been able to DO a thing for my patient. I poured out my whole, sad story. She just stood there with her Mona Lisa smile, listening patiently, nodding as she allowed me to ramble and cry. Then she took my hand and spoke.

"You don't have to DO anything, Mary Rives. Go back to her

16

room and sit on the side of the bed ("Oh my God. Sit on the side of the bed? But, but, but, but we're **never** supposed to sit on the side of the bed!" My thoughts screamed in my head). Take her hand and hold it and don't try to say or DO anything. Just sit there, be with her, and allow her to grieve and to cry. Give her your quiet concern and support because she needs that more than she needs for you to bathe her or change her bed."

I returned to my patient's room with the warmth of Mrs. Brown's advice draping my shoulders, giving me the strength to enter and sit quietly on the side of her bed as she cried. Tears slipped down my cheeks and landed in my lap as hers dampened her pillow. We sat for what seemed ages, holding hands. She looked up, let go of my hand, and reached over to her bedside table to pick up a fistful of tissues. Rubbing her back and tucking her in, no words ever exchanged; I pulled up the rail and went to my post-clinical conference.

As we sat in the conference room sharing the events of our day, I dreaded the point when I would speak because my experience was uneventful. However, I felt it was the heart and soul of what nursing is supposed to be. Maybe, just maybe, there was more to all of this DOING than I thought. The doing was the mechanics of nursing. The quiet concern and support, the caring, the life-affirming beliefs within each of my fellow nurses—this was the energy and the basis for all that we were to accomplish in our careers. How in the world was I to share all that was going on in my mind?

Then, as if someone had known what I was thinking, the door opened and the charge nurse from the obstetrical ward stuck her head in the room and beckoned Mrs. Brown. Both of them looked at me and my heart stopped. Mrs. Brown walked quietly over to me and whispered in my ear that I was to leave and return to my patient's bedside and she'd be there to collect me when our clinical was over.

I rushed to my patient's room, fearing everything. Did the baby die? Did I do something wrong? Did my patient hemorrhage? Did they see the imprint of my behind on the side of the bed?

Opening her door, I slipped in to find her sitting up in bed with the blinds open, sunlight streaming in. Flowers and greeting cards surrounded her. Smiling, she said, "I just wanted to say thank you for sitting with me this morning. I was feeling so very helpless because my baby and my husband and family weren't here with me. I wasn't even allowed to bathe myself or go to the bathroom. I was not in control of anything—my baby's birth or my own body—and all I could do was cry. But you stopped trying to control everything for me and just allowed me to cry. You gave me the one thing I needed more than anything else in the world, and that was your personal concern about what I was feeling while everyone around me was telling me to keep a stiff upper lip and go about the business of healing from childbirth. My husband just called and told me that our baby is doing well and when I'm discharged, he will come pick me up and take me to a hotel near the hospital so that I can see him. Nothing that has happened so far in this whole experience has affected me as strongly as that phone call and your help this morning."

I never forgot that day. It has been a day that has been replayed thousands of times in the past 20 years. The faces are different, situations may be different, and the outcome may not always be as positive, but in that moment with Mrs. Brown in the hallway two decades ago, I learned one of the biggest, most profound lessons I will ever learn.

A Hospice Death

Ann Lederer

Early in the evening of one of my first nights on call as a hospice nurse, I tried to ignore the sense of foreboding creeping in. My day had been unusual, as most of the nurses had been at a workshop. Because any situation out of the ordinary (such as a thunderstorm or losing a basketball game) had the potential for setting off a flurry of calls, I was certain they were coming, so I waited. I decided to boost my immune system with a quick walk before the inevitable happened. Almost as if by schedule, the calls started coming, but I was not prepared for the gift I was to receive in the disguise of an urgent call that one of our patients had died.

I raced to the neighborhood already familiar to me, although I was new to this town. My patient's street had quite a reputation—crack houses, drug busts, a tragic fire, you name it. Having worked in Detroit at an AIDS clinic, I prided myself on my fearlessness and openness to cultural diversity, but as I circled the dim street hunting for a house number and parking space, a group of boys appeared out of nowhere, startling me. I reached for my cellular phone and dialed my patient's home number. The line was busy. I pulled into a neighbor's driveway and placed my stethoscope around my neck, a symbol to the neighborhood that I was a nurse—here to help, not harm. Quickly, I stepped to the front door and knocked.

The tiny house was packed with people. Led to the center room, I found a ring of people encircling the bed, and as I approached, they stepped aside. They watched me silently as I put the stethoscope to her heart and felt her wrist for pulses. Skin still warm, she appeared to be sleeping. I thought I should continue checking for signs of life a little longer. It was my duty to pronounce her dead, and I was struck with awe at this responsibility. Wrapping the blood pressure cuff around her upper arm and pumping it with air, I mumbled, "Just a formality." Someone nodded politely.

She was a small, frail, elderly woman, about my mother's age. I did not know the details of her illness, as she had been under another nurse's care, but I did know what to do and say from this point on. She was my patient tonight, and I quickly stepped into my role. "Have you decided on a funeral home? I can call them now if you are ready." Some wept, some prayed, and some got on the telephone and called more people. Quickly, the house filled to overflowing—a small house consisting of only three tiny rooms.

As we waited for the mortician, some members of the crowd became individuals. The patient's exhausted husband. The oldest daughter, who had made the call to me. The youngest child who now held his mother's hands, sobbing. Various great grandchildren. The Pastor. Two elderly white ladies, a definite minority in this sea of dark-skinned faces.

In between tears, the family pieced together my patient's story. She had been a little more restless than usual. Her husband lay down on the bed next to her and began to pray. She relaxed. Her breathing eased, then stopped. They called the hospice nurse on call, as planned. They had nothing but praise for their hospice team. I reminded them of the beautiful gift they had given her—the gift of being allowed to die in her own home.

As the funeral home staff arrived, I watched as the crowd parted. "This part can be very difficult," I said, "You might not want to watch." I tried counting heads and stopped around forty. The praying, which had been very soft, now crescendoed into a wave of harmonies. There was no longer loud crying, but there were tears. The praying continued for several minutes after the hearse drove off. As I began collecting my things, I paid my respects again. A son walked me to my car, and as I looked around, I noticed no parking spaces were available on the whole block.

Later reflecting on this event, I realized how privileged I had been to glimpse a part of their lives during this death. I felt embarrassed for dreading the night on call, especially for my worries about safety. The image of all the family members and close friends supporting each other at this sad time uplifted me. Inspired by the sound of music so foreign to my ears, only a neighborhood away, I was moved to tell this story.

My Little Greek Friend

Kathy Lilleby

Every year at Christmas, I think of my little Greek patient as I hang the ornament that he gave me on my tree. But, that wasn't the only gift I received from that brave little boy.

I was a nurse on a pediatric bone marrow transplant unit when I was asked to care for Billy, an eight-year-old boy of Greek descent. The first time I walked into his room, I felt he and I were an unlikely match. I related better to toddlers and teenage girls. What was I going to do with an eight-year-old boy? At first, the only way I connected with him was through his Hickman catheter since I had to use it to draw so many blood samples and administer medications.

But after a few days, we fell into a routine, and began to feel more comfortable with each other. I discovered that one sure way to get him to take medicine or get out of bed and walk was to give him a back scratch. He loved it, and it worked every time!

Billy soon contracted a fungal infection and required daily doses of Amphotericin B (nicknamed "Shake and Bake"). To prevent the ensuing chills and fever that accompany this type of therapy, I gave pre-medications through his catheter. Since it took a while to slowly push them and then flush the line with saline, he would ask me to scratch his back while we were waiting. By this time, the back scratch had become a way for me to comfort him while his mother was home for a break.

While I was sitting on the edge of the bed and scratching Billy's back one evening, he asked, "Kathy, you know what?" "No, what?" I replied. "You're my friend," he said. My eyes filling with tears, I was unable to say a word with the large lump that formed in my throat. What other words could have been more special to me? I realized that Billy and I had truly become friends.

He died a few weeks later, just before Christmas. Our special friendship lives with me to this day.

The Blizzard and The Flood

Barbara A. Brown

I was a small child in 1941, the year of the Armistice Day Blizzard in South Dakota. During this terrible blizzard, my appendix ruptured, and knowing that this was a medical emergency best handled by specialists, my family doctor made arrangements for a snow plow to create a safe path to the nearest large hospital about 25 miles away. My father drove me to the hospital with the family doctor in the back seat with me. I had the surgery and recovered in the hospital for about six weeks (these were the days before antibiotics and sulfa drugs). When I think back on this event, I believe it's a miracle I survived.

Thirty-one years later, in 1972, Rapid City, on the far western edge of our state, suffered a killer flood. Hundreds of lives were lost, and all persons with medical or nursing training were called to work. I found myself called in on special duty to help care for a patient who came all the way to Sioux Falls to have surgery for a fractured wrist. Now, why would someone come 400 miles in the middle of a natural disaster to our Sioux Falls hospital for treatment for something as minor as a fractured wrist? I discovered that the patient was the same physician who had seen me through the blizzard trip so long ago.

He had retired in Rapid City, and when he fell and broke his wrist, he was too thoughtful to burden the local medical community in Rapid City with this trivial concern, so he decided to charter a plane, return to Sioux Falls, and receive the medical treatment he needed. I reminded him who I was, and we both marveled at this coincidence that had brought us together again in time of a natural disaster--but, this time I was the one helping him!

The Love of God

Lenore Lang

"Please Ma. Make you come quick-quick!" Through our open front door, I looked into the face of an African woman. Behind her on the verandah were four other people. A quick glance showed no sick child with them. So, what would be the problem? A bad accident somewhere? A case of malaria in one of the homes? A woman in labor? In the year and a half since our arrival, these were the types of situations that we often encountered. But today was going to be somewhat different, as I was soon to discover.

"Now whattee?" I asked in my hesitant Pidgin English, which was slowly improving over the weeks as I communicated with my Limbum-speaking friends at the Bible School where my husband was Principal and Tutor. "Nah, some woman..." the story unfolded. Friends had carried a pregnant woman a great distance, and she was in a house across the road from our African mission compound. They needed my help now!

My medicine box was waiting--bandages, scissors, and White Cross materials generously donated by Christian women back in the States. Supplies in hand, we quickly passed through the Mission gate and crossed the road as I marveled at the simple trust these people had that this missionary wife, nurse, and mother could "make it better."

I reflected on the long distance these friends had carried the woman, looking for help. Cars, trucks, lorries, and Land Rovers were few and far between. In fact, the only vehicle for miles around was right here on our Mission compound, and my husband was the only driver. So, if it meant a trip to our Mission hospital 20 miles down the road, he would be the one behind the wheel.

Maybe it wouldn't come to that. Maybe I'd be able to deliver the baby without complications. "Please, Lord, help me," I silently prayed.

Inside the house, I was shocked to discover the extent of the trust these people had in me. The woman had delivered a child feet first with the head still in the birth canal. What pain and trauma this woman had already endured, along with the pain of knowing that her child was dead.

Somehow I managed to extricate the head from the birth canal. Stoically, the mother accepted the pain. Next, I felt her abdomen to estimate the size of the placenta. Soon, it was time to deliver the placenta. There it came, sliding out--but wait! This was no ordinary placenta, surely! It was--could it be? There were membranes surrounding a live child!

Quickly, I tore away the membranes. The infant gasped and began to cry. A son! The women who were helping me cried out in joy, with the patient joining in. A weak and tired new mother was ecstatic.

As I left the house with a thankful heart, the Limbum name of the child rang in my ears. What was that name, which the mother gave almost immediately to her new son? Kong-nyu, meaning "The Love of God." A wonderful name, expressing the joy of us all!

Shades of White

Tee Angel

It has been a long road to this point. The university was a protected and sacred place. Now, I am learning at an accelerated rate: circumstances are ever changing. To say that speed is of the essence is to understate. In the hospital, people come and go so quickly. My skills are newly acquired, my knowledge broad and unapplied, so I go in many directions in my head. What to do first, when, and why—all a jumble of organizational muck. My first days are full of questions to which I have no immediate answers. Are special relationships with my patients possible, or was that just something they told us in school?

Starting my nursing practice felt more like being shot out of a cannon than I ever would have imagined. My floor is a fast-paced telemetry unit. "Surely this feeling will pass," I thought, "this sense of overwhelming inadequacy, even fear." Well, I was wrong. It did not happen that I suddenly felt superbly proficient. I did not immediately become organized, or have planned and allotted time to simply "be" with my patients. Instead, I enter into a room filled with shades of white; my nursing practice became all I wanted within the passing of a single moment.

She is tiny, and oh so frail in a hospital bed three sizes too big for her frame. Her hair is tangled, in complete disarray. She looks up at me as though she has known me all her life, reaches for my hand, and pulls me down beside her. I stroke her hand and we simply sit for what seems like an immeasurable amount of time without speaking. In those few seconds, I have completely come to know her and she knows me. We are partners in the events that will begin one life as another passes.

As I introduce myself, she smiles from deep inside herself and the spirit of a giant is unleashed before me. We talk as I assess her—heart, lungs, pulses. The years have not been kind. Too much alcohol and tobacco are claiming their due. But at this stage, at this age, what right have I, a spectator, to judge her lived experience? I have not shared her joys, sorrows, accomplishments, and defeats.

I learn that she has a joy of life and being that many have never experienced. Driving her car, going out to play bridge, shopping, eating out. Her days are full and happy. Then, she awoke only 48 hours ago with paralysis of her right side, and too weak to walk. This is how I came to meet her. Tired, too sore to move, her right arm clutched tightly to her side with decreased circulation to that hand. Yet, her mind is as clear and succinct as anyone I know. Her gift of humor could lighten anyone's day.

I went in and out of her room a dozen times that morning. By afternoon, we were well acquainted and the conversations picked up immediately where they'd left off. But, her assessments were increasingly troubling. There had been a subtle change in skin color by shift's end. I left report that day and went in to say good night. We sat talking, quietly, laughing over stories of her past, ending with the promise that I'd return in the morning. Shades of white had dimmed in the dusk.

The morning came as promised, and I greeted the day with more confidence than I had felt during the previous weeks. I received report, learning that my patients had fared well during the night. No changes, no emergencies, nothing missed: all is well. I have the same group and feel that I know my patients well. Assessments done, medications supplied, the morning moves at a brisk pace. Yet I feel equipped to handle the pace—knowing my patients and having them know me makes all the difference. Trust has been established.

I have come to bathe her, my tiny one. Time for daily weight—close attention to skin, circulation, strength, coordination—all the many things we check in a moment's observation. The unending list of things to do, sometimes clouding the vision of care. I run the water, bring the supplies, pull the drapes. There is no pretense between us: I have come to do more than bathe her. I am here to be with her. She talks of her life and shares herself with me. Her family relationships are constrained by feelings of loss and abandonment. A single parent, she did the best she could. We worked together to clean away the hurt and come to a place of acceptance. I put lotion on her skin, softening the dryness and comforting her heart. I touch her to give care and assistance that transcend intent to meet her many needs. She is no longer alone. Her hair is done, her spirits are rejuvenated. Explaining that her hand is a growing concern, we initiate a plan of care.

The consults are called—cardiac physician calls surgical physician to assess. It is the end of the shift and suddenly all events are coming to a head. I give report and return to her bedside. The quiet solitude we experienced has been replaced with many new faces and lots of them. A surgeon stands on one side, a cardiac specialist on the other. Daughter and granddaughter are there. The tension and pressure are on. A demand to make a decision weighs heavily in the air. The medical team advises surgery to open the arm to remove an extensive blood clot. The vision of a speeding train comes to mind. She is tied to the tracks with no escape. Any decision leads her to a place where she does not wish to be. The shades of white have turned to black.

The cardiologist states that a week ago she was living a full life. The surgeon maintains that without surgery, she will die. With surgery, she will probably lose her arm. Surviving the operation is not guaranteed. Renal failure, which she has, is not reversible. Her heart is weak. There is a 20% chance she'll keep the arm and tolerate the surgery. She looks up at me and reaches for my hand.

"This can't be happening. I feel like I'm on a game show trying to pick the right door. The problem is…there is no right door." She is clear and concise about her desire not to live without her arm. There is an understanding that her life will never be the same and that either choice is a step toward ending her time here. They are pushing her on many sides. Physicians urge quick and aggressive action. No time to think. The train picks up speed.

Everyone leaves the room to confer in the hallway. I lag behind and sit close to her. No words need be said. I have no desire to push her in any direction. I wish her only peace. She smiles a slow, even smile, "I'm going to die either way. I want to go out the way I came in, in one piece. I don't want to have to look around for parts of my body as I leave this world." I nod understanding of her joking words, knowing she is making the choice from her heart. She suddenly realizes I am here past my shift and asks, "Why?" To be with her. "Go home. I'll be all right and I'll see you tomorrow. I'm not going anywhere tonight," she says. I look back as I leave the room. She smiles and waves, then blows me a kiss, which I return. Shades of gray reflect in the setting sun from her room.

I don't know what made me call the ward that night. Some inner thought or need to say good night, I guess. The night nurse said that my patient had been taken to surgery shortly after I left. The family had signed the consent, feeling she was not clear enough to make the decision. There was no news yet, but everything would work out fine.

Night turns to day. When I return to the hospital, she is foremost in my thoughts. She is no longer on the floor. I inquire about her at the desk. The operation did not go well. The arm was lost—her heart and respirations failed on the operating table. She was intubated, stabilized, and moved to critical care. There would be no recovery.

Stillness came settling in, surrounding my thoughts, bringing quiet, nothing more. Later that morning the surgeon stopped in to say he had a message for the nurse who cared for "the woman" he operated on last night. As she was prepped for surgery, she had looked up into his eyes, reached for his hand, and said, "Tell my nurse I love her." The anesthesia took over. Those were to be her last words.

During lunch I went to see her. She had been restless, even in her unconscious state. Her vital signs were unstable and failing. The place where her arm used to be was heavily bandaged and awkward on her small frame. It was time, and I had come to say good-bye. Taking her hand in mine, bending close to her ear, I spoke the words within my heart. "I love you too, my friend. Good-bye." I kissed her cheek and feel sure she squeezed my hand. She was gone within the hour.

There are many days I think of her. Her funny laugh and love of life, the way she allowed me into her world. A living, shared experience where I still find her in all the colors of the rainbow, knowing I will always treasure the gift she gave me, wrapped in the most incredible shades of white.

Whose Call Is It?

Susan Roisen

"They are bringing down John Doe. They found him on the floor at the nursing home. We need to do a full resuscitation and he should be here right now."

The nurse hangs up the phone, the elevator doors open and there they are. John on the gurney, a nurse, and two assistants: all desperately attempting to keep their patient breathing. His face is as blue as the waters of the Caribbean.

Into the cardiac unit they wheel him. Nurses hook up monitors and oxygen. Intravenous lines are placed in every available vein, and fluids are running in rapidly. The medical doctor arrives.

"Does he have a pulse? Did anyone witness this?" He places a breathing tube down the patient's trachea. "Does anyone have a stethoscope? Listen to his chest for air," he asks. Cardiopulmonary resuscitation continues, and John does not respond. We administer medications to help his heart beat, and then we defibrillate. Fifty minutes have passed quickly. John's wife arrives in a wheelchair, followed by her granddaughter-in-law in tears. "You've got to wake up, Pa," she pleads as she caresses his hand.

"Cora, do you want us to continue?" the doctor asks his wife. "Yes, I want to keep him forever!" she answers, as she wheels herself out of the room. "Please do whatever you can."

The priest enters and gives last rites. His is a comforting presence. We continue CPR another 10 minutes, and then we stop. Our resuscitation has failed. The physician leaves, feeling defeated. The nurses attend to the body, relieved. Nursing home staff return to their duties, drained of emotion.

Cora returns to say her last good-byes. "Why did you have to leave me, Pa?" she cries. The priest comes into the room, and the three are left alone. Cora and the priest kneel and pray. The almighty presence

29

of God the Father enters the room, along with a quiet peace. John is taken from Cora and placed in the loving arms of Jesus and ushered into heaven.

With all our technology, all our devoted love, affection, and care, there is only one who has the final call.

Naked Cora

Beth Flanagan

When I tell people I work in a nursing home, they almost always say, "That must be depressing." There are things about nursing home work that are emotionally trying, such as watching some of my patients live in a vegetative state day after day, lying in whatever position until someone comes in to turn them over. It's sad to see residents whose families stop coming to visit because they are unable to cope with a parent who no longer recognizes them. Yet almost every day, something happens that reminds me how much I am needed, and I can honestly say that my job is far from depressing, like having a resident grab onto my arm to keep from falling, or seeing tired old eyes look into mine and thank me for a drink of water after a nap. It also makes me appreciate my own life a little more when I see pictures of them when they were my age. "They were once like me," I think to myself.

Cora Hayden was one of those residents who made me ask myself on several occasions what I was thinking when I decided to become a nurse. She had been with us for six months and had kept us hopping the whole time. So far, she had socked two nurses' aides and managed to wrestle a shot away from the 11-7 nurse and chase her around the desk with it. Recently, she broke up the staff appreciation party early when she walked in in all her naked glory and gave the administrator a cursing out. To say she was confused would have been putting it mildly.

Today, as I began my rounds, Cora tugged at my sleeve. "Hey, girl. Do you have a knife? Let me have it. I want to go home," she said as she nervously glanced around the room. Her lipstick was smeared across her face, and she had one high heel on with a house slipper. "I'm going to get that boy who tricked me into coming here. One of these days I'm going to kill him." Obviously, Cora was her usual self today. She was always threatening to kill some boy but when we asked her who it was, she would only stare at us a bit and say she didn't know. I told her I

31

didn't have a knife, to which she replied, "Well, shit!" as she shook her fist at me. "Bring it to my room. That's what I pay you to do!" Then she took off down the hallway by herself.

A few minutes later, I was helping the aides with their evening duties by passing out trays. When I took Cora's to her, I found her lying on her bed, staring out the window. I set her tray down and began picking up pictures that I supposed she'd dropped on the floor. One of them caught my attention. It looked like it had been taken sometime in the 70's, judging by the way the people were dressed. In the middle of the family photo stood a graceful-looking woman of about 40, holding a pink bundle in her arms. I picked up another picture off the floor and saw that it was of Cora and her husband, Jim. She stood behind him in this photo, her hand resting on his shoulder, his large hand nearly swallowing hers in their embrace. Jim died two weeks after Cora came to the nursing home. Her daughter said he'd had a massive heart attack out in the fields by himself. Cora had never asked about him. We assumed she didn't know what was going on.

As I handed the pictures to her, she motioned to the table and said, "Take that stuff away. I don't want anything to eat. I'm too tired." That struck me as odd because she always ate everything that she wasn't testing the laws of gravity with. When I asked her if I could check her blood pressure and temperature, she grabbed my arm and pulled me down to her. Fearing a beating, I resisted, but she pulled again. "I'm going somewhere, girl," she said. "I want you to watch the house for me. I won't be gone long," she said. I told her I would, then left her alone.

When I clocked in a few days later, I noticed that a voice was absent among the noise of call bells, phones, and the hustle of the day shift trying to get done. "I know what's missing," I thought to myself, "Cora." I learned in report that Cora had starting feeling bad at about six o'clock Saturday morning, complaining of a headache, and behaving lethargically. Her vital signs were normal, however.

I went to her room first. She was asleep and her expression was one of a person in a peaceful dream. She was smiling a half smile, and she moaned softly as I checked her blood pressure. I whispered to her to hang in there, and she moved her foot and opened her eyes slightly.

Around 6 PM, one of the aides called me to Cora's room. She wanted to get up, so we combed her hair, put her glasses on, and dressed her in a light blue robe and gown. She pulled herself up holding onto the siderail, and motioned, "T.V." We took her to the activity room.

About an hour later, I passed by there, and noticed that another resident had put a rose in Cora's blonde hair. She looked absolutely radiant!

The beauty of the moment ended when Cora let out a mournful wail then slumped over in her wheelchair, unresponsive. We took her back to her room once and checked her vitals, noting that they had dropped markedly. Cora's physician was notified, and the orders were simple: keep her comfortable. Earlier in the disease process, when she could still make decisions for herself, Cora had indicated that she didn't want any heroic measures should anything happen.

I contacted her daughter and told her about the change in her mother's condition. She said she would try to call her brother. I didn't know Cora had a son.

The night dragged on with Cora fighting every minute for life. Cora was always hardheaded, and this was no different. Death calls and Cora tells him to wait a darn minute. She had taken on a gray appearance and her cheeks sank inward with every breath. Her pulse was 38 beats a minute. We dimmed the lights in her room, and held her hands. I didn't care what was going on outside this room; my only concern was not letting her die alone.

Cora took a deep breath and held it, slowly exhaled, and stopped breathing. She continued this for several minutes. I knew what she was waiting for.

When her children arrived, the son was the first to speak. "I'm sorry, Mother," he said before starting to cry. The daughter reached for his hand and said, "Bill, it's o.k. Mom knew what was happening to her. That's why she had you get her a living will." Both of them were holding her hands. As Cora gasped her last breaths, her daughter whispered to her, "We're going to miss you, Momma. Tell Daddy we said Hi," as she kissed Cora on the forehead. "You two can pick up where you left off." With those words in her ear, Cora took her last breath. She was 61 years old.

Thank You, Aunt Tommie

Paula Schneider

Recently, as I was going through some old photographs, I ran across a picture of myself with Aunt Tommie in my grandmother's back yard. I was seven years old then, all decked out in a costume of nursing cap and cape. Aunt Tommie beamed proudly down at me. That photograph reminded me of the advice my aunt gave me all those years ago and how it affected my life.

Aunt Tommie epitomized the stately matriarch with her thick, silver hair held in a French twist with beaded combs she made herself. Visiting her in San Antonio, Texas as a child, I joined her in the kitchen as she cooked squash, our favorite vegetable. "Paula, your health is the most important thing in your life," she said. "If you don't have good health, you don't have anything."

As a teenager in the 1960s and 1970s, I again thought about her words of advice to me—words that, I believe, prevented me from experimenting with drugs and cigarettes. I simply did not want to do anything to cause possible harm to my body, even though all of my acquaintances and most of my friends were wildly trying new ways of altering reality.

Later, as an adult, I decided on a career as a nurse. Over the past 20+ years as a nurse, I have shared Aunt Tommie's philosophy of health with patients and co-workers. I attracted a wonderful husband with a degree in health education, and together we do our best to live and to model health for others. We get plenty of rest, eat a low-fat, mostly vegetarian diet, exercise as much as possible, and surround ourselves with supportive friends and family. Together we have created peaceful and fulfilling lives.

The health profession has allowed me to grow personally, continue to learn how to live healthily, and to share valuable information with others so that they, too, might enjoy the rewards of healthy lifestyles.

This has been most rewarding for me, and I revel in the richness of it each time I see people benefit from the information I am able to give them.

Easing Her Pain

Carol Lewis

Although most of my nursing experience has been in the field of adult, chronic pain management, I recently was called upon to work with Sara, an infant only five days old who had undergone major thoracic surgery. As I looked at this frail, new body that weighed no more than six pounds, I was shaking in my boots. She had a tube protruding from every available orifice, her legs were drawn up, and I could see the pain on her face. She was fighting for her life!

My thought was, "I know adult pain management, not pediatric." So, after reviewing the orders at least three times and rechecking the dosages more than a dozen times, I went to work. Viewing her tiny body one more time, I suddenly felt a sense of purpose and a reaching out for my expertise. Even though she was unable to talk to me, a powerful message came from her to me that night. I knew I was needed.

I prepared her special pain medication pump and proceeded to dose her catheter. Within 15 minutes, she was beginning to relax, her vital signs were returning to normal, and her little legs slackened into a normal position. She required two more doses of pain medication that night, and rested comfortably.

Knowing I had made a difference in this little one's life gave me a rush of satisfaction that was extremely fulfilling. Sara was a fighter, and made a speedy recovery. She left the hospital three days after surgery. Even though I played a small part in her total care, I was renewed in my commitment to pain management. This is what brings me back to work day after day. Though ultimate outcomes are sometimes beyond our control, we can make a difference in our patients' lives.

Viola's Choice

Maria Schulz

Viola made her choice. Her mother, Elsie, a sweet, grey-haired, petite lady with sparkling, sky-blue eyes, was ready to come home from the hospital. Viola and her three sisters debated their options. Should they place 89-year-old Elsie in a nursing home so she could obtain the around-the-clock help she would need with eating, dressing, bathing, and managing her Foley catheter? Or would it be best to bring her home and let Viola care for her? These were just two of the many options discussed, but Viola knew what she wanted to do.

Viola, the oldest of the four sisters, was 71 years old herself. She and her mother had shared a home together for the past 30 years. Home was where Elsie belonged, and Viola wanted to care for her mother herself. With the decision made, Viola sought out the help of the home health agency and the hospital, who worked together to ensure everything Elsie would need, such as a hospital bed and medical supplies, were in place when she arrived home from the hospital.

I was lucky enough to be the registered nurse assigned to Mrs. Elsie Gray. My first meeting with her not only centered around performing a physical assessment, but also getting details of Elsie's past medical history, the medications she was currently taking, and just getting to know the family's needs related to Elsie's care. I made arrangements for a home health aide, Suzie, to visit three times a week to provide Elsie's personal care, and also for a social worker to assess the situation to see if she qualified for any other assistance. Viola had already qualified for some respite services, and Michelle came two days a week so Viola could have some time for herself.

At first, I visited three times a week in order to teach Viola how to care for her mother's Foley catheter. I also taught her the basics of skin care, the need for frequent turning, and how to improve her mother's nutrition. Viola had very good instincts about caring for a bedbound patient, and was an excellent caregiver. She learned quickly. The only drawback was her physical endurance and the fact that she was on duty for her mother 24 hours a day. We made sure Viola took care of herself as well as her mother.

As any home care nurse will tell you, a very special bond develops when we visit a patient so frequently. I looked forward to my visits with Elsie and Viola. I enjoyed helping celebrate Elsie's 90th birthday, and fondly remember my visits in December when Elsie's coverlet on her bed was a bright, cheery Christmas scene.

Physical therapists tried to help Elsie regain her strength so she could get out of bed for short trips in a wheelchair, but they were unsuccessful. Elsie could not tolerate much activity without experiencing chest pain or a drop in her blood pressure. Viola slowly came to the realization that her mother's health was failing and that she would be bedbound for the rest of her life.

Around that time, Viola presented her mother with a canary. The canary lived in a cage at the foot of Elsie's bed. Now, Elsie's days were filled with bursts of sound by her songbird, and it seemed to me that as Elsie grew weaker, the canary sang even more beautifully.

Elsie grew more listless and her weakened heart began to fail. Our goal was to keep her as comfortable as possible. An air mattress on her bed, meticulous care by Michelle, Suzie, and Viola, high-calorie foods and milk shakes, and ongoing social worker and nursing support all helped to make Elsie's final days comfortable. Viola tired very easily, dealing with the physical rigors of caring for her mother while working through the dynamics of slowly allowing her mother to go.

As Elsie grew weaker and less able to talk, Viola and her sisters discussed whether Elsie would want to be admitted to the hospital when she seemed near death. Viola insisted Elsie would wish to remain at home, and her sisters agreed. One day in March, I got the call I had been expecting. Elsie was unable to eat or drink, and was barely responsive. When I arrived at her home, I found the house filled with the four daughters and their families who were there to be supportive.

Elsie lived a few days longer. Soon the room only held an empty hospital bed and the canary. Even he mourned her passing, for he abruptly ceased his song and lost his feathers.

Viola and I still keep in touch. Her determination and will to help her mother through her last days, with dignity and in familiar surroundings, was truly courageous. The canary resumed his song and has grown new feathers. The hospital bed is gone, along with the supplies. But Elsie's dresser, full of her belongings, stays untouched. I think this is Viola's way of still keeping Elsie at home, with her, in the place they both loved and shared.

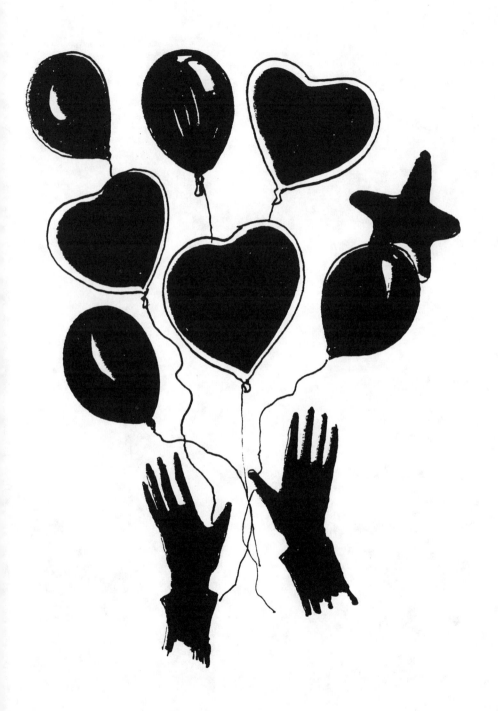

2

Breaking the Illusion

Some experiences of nurses cannot be easily described in everyday terms. As we attempt to find explanations for sensations, feelings, and intuitions, we often come to a brick wall. But, even though we may not know why these things happen or what they mean, these events occur nonetheless.

Continue reading for some interesting tales from nurses who have been brushed by angel wings and have had other types of fascinating, often unexplained, experiences.

Angel in the Black Robe

Lavon Lockwood

Our patient was a young, Hispanic girl of nine or ten years who was admitted to the hospital because of headaches and loss of vision. A CAT scan of the brain detected a tumor, and even though her physicians suspected it was not malignant, when removed, would leave her permanently blind. The pediatric staff was very upset with this news, as was the family.

The night before the surgery, our charge nurse spoke with the child, who was being very brave about the whole ordeal. During the evening hours, a priest came in to visit another patient. Since we live in a city with a large Catholic population, it is not at all unusual to see unfamiliar clergy in the hospital halls. The charge nurse requested that the priest visit with the child and her family and he said he would. He went to see the first child briefly, visited our patient, and then wished the charge nurse a good evening as he exited the ward.

After he left, the charge nurse went in to see our young, stoic patient, who said to the nurse, "I really like your smock. It's so pretty." The little girl assured the nurse she was able to see it, and that she especially liked the pink color. The nurse, acting in her most therapeutic, but grounded, manner, countered with a firm statement that it was time to stop pretending. But the little girl persisted, and was further able to identify objects in the room accurately!

We quickly called the child's physician, who cancelled the surgery and discharged our patient the next morning.

Our brave little patient told us that the "nice father" had come in to her room, prayed with her, and then with her sight restored, told her he was glad she felt better and to get a good night's sleep. Upon checking around, we discovered that the parents of the first child had no idea who the priest was—they just assumed their parish had sent him. No one, to our knowledge, ever found out the priest's name.

Visiting Hours

Michael Worley

In 1994, I was working in a rural town, halfway between Denver and Cheyenne. The size and number of family-owned farms were shrinking yearly, and the fields of red-tasseled wheat were replaced by new homes for swarming California emigrants. The native inhabitants and their culture were taking a little longer to be removed. Only the Rocky Mountains, towering 50 miles to the west, were too big to be bulldozed and platted.

Our 75-bed general hospital served the people of the surrounding plains, where many of the small towns had already marked their centennial. Dry farming on the eastern slope of the mountains had been a gamble before modern water projects. Crops might fail without warning and herds die wholesale in unexpected droughts, wiping out the fortunes of entire towns, as well as families' livelihoods. In this uncertain world, men and women were raised to rely on one another far more than in wetter climates. And when someone—a child, mother, or father— became ill and was hospitalized, family members could be expected to visit at any time. Frequently, adult children would pick up an infirm patient who could no longer drive, allowing them a chance to visit an ill spouse at our hospital. Few ever missed a chance to be at the bedside of a sick husband or wife, to watch television, share news of home, or just sit quietly together.

Sometimes it was hard to distinguish some of these fragile, elderly visitors from their hospitalized spouses. We'd take two sets of vital signs instead of one and make sure the visitor had eaten more than a cold sandwich for lunch, and in the evening, we sometimes bedded them down on a cot in the same room. Many retired couples still lived and managed a little house by themselves while being checked on daily by their grown children or a friendly neighbor. We marveled at their ability to live independently and admired their mutual devotion, which was as plain and tangible as their gold wedding bands. At home, they kept track of each other's medications, managed the difficult transfers from bed to wheelchair and back to bed again, gave daily sponge baths and back rubs, and managed the cooking and cleaning—a routine of tasks that would daunt people half their age. And finally, when a mate died despite their devoted care, the one left behind was generally also buried within a year's time.

The Markheims, Margaret and Larry, had been married for 52 years. Seventy and 68 years old, their lives could have resembled any of a hundred couples who came to our hospital each year. She, with multiple sclerosis, hypothyroidism, multiple strokes, and a myriad of lesser problems, was hospitalized about every two to three months to have her health stabilized and medications changed. This last admission came after Larry stopped some of her medications without consulting their doctor when he saw his wife in more than her usual pain. Margaret, initially with an unstable blood pressure, was now improving after four days of supervised medical care. Larry greeted her every day at sunrise, despite his own history of heart problems that interfered with his breathing and energy levels. But, despite his own discomfort, he kept watch in her room every day, his swollen ankles propped up on a bedside chair, all the while smiling and holding Margaret's hand.

For many reasons, we were grateful for his presence. Margaret, suffering from mild dementia, became restless when left alone, refused to eat, and remained sleepless at night. When Larry was with her, she was transformed. Fed from his hand, she would eat heartily; we always made sure he had a tray of his own so they could share their mealtimes. Her twitching face would smooth as she calmed and smiled.

Though unable to keep a fresh thought in mind for more than five minutes, Margaret became able to speak and recall minute details of their married life from years ago. Having seen much of America by rail in their younger days, they would sit together and remember, as if they were still passengers on a train. Their afternoons were spent rolling through that beloved and familiar country of their lives, pointing out the landmarks to one another as they passed. The trip was so real to them, the memories so alive and fresh, that the nurses could get lost in their room for hours. Margaret and Larry were together every day, from dawn to sundown, in a never-ending journey.

One morning Larry failed to show up for breakfast. Early morning

43

became late morning. Margaret refused to eat despite much coaxing and started to become restless. This unexplained absence was unlike Larry, and we became concerned. We called their house many times, but he never answered. Shortly after noon, Margaret began calling out his name louder and louder and refused to be consoled.

At 1:00 PM that afternoon, we received a phone call from Chuck, Larry and Margaret's eldest son. He had found Larry in the kitchen next to the stove. He had been dead for several hours. Chuck cried as he told us of his father's death, and said he and the rest of the family would be at the hospital shortly to break the news to Margaret.

Meanwhile, about the time of Chuck's call, Margaret became silent. Unresponsive, we called her doctor and then lifted her back to bed. Her blood pressure was low, and we started intravenous fluids. Her vital signs continued to slowly decline, and by 1:30 PM when her children arrived, her condition was very serious. We told the family of her condition, and with the physician, decided to make her a "No Code" before telling her of Larry's death, fully expecting the news to kill her.

Her children never got the chance to tell her about Larry. Their mother's blood pressure and heart rate continued to gently, steadily fall, like a bit of chaff on still air. With her family gathered in the room, Margaret's heart finally stopped at 2:17 that afternoon. She never regained consciousness.

Margaret and Larry were buried four days later, side by side, in a little cemetery beside a prairie lake, the water reflecting the blue of the cloudless sky overhead. Their story was discussed for many weeks, especially by the night staff. It has become one of our hospital's legends. We pass it on to certain newcomers, but not all.

When a difficult death is in the works, an agony whose length seems to serve no purpose, when another couple is about to be parted, we remember the Markheims. We remember their love and their devotion to each other, which transcends illness, time, and perhaps death itself.

On frosty winter nights you can hear the Union-Pacific's whistle as it passes through our little town and nearly all the way to Cheyenne. Its regularity reminds us of Larry's promise to visit Margaret. You see, many of us believe that Larry managed to keep his promise that day, and that they left together to continue, somehow, their never-ending journey.

Sam and Eva

Tricia Cooke

After 63 years together, it took a hospitalization to separate Sam and Eva Windsor. Married at age 17 despite objections from both families, they weathered many stormy periods together. They had raised two sons to manhood, celebrated when both married, and basked in the loving attention from their grandchildren. The wedding anniversary party had started off wonderfully on a beautiful May day. Every single member of their family had managed to gather for this happy occasion. Sadly, gaiety and laughter dissolved into tears as Eva misjudged the height of the steps leading off the dance floor and fell helplessly to the ground. Sam had been walking directly behind Eva and had almost fallen himself in a desperate attempt to protect Eva. Eva barely called out as the pain shot through her left hip. "Oh, Sam!" she cried, "I've ruined the party." "Hush, hush sweetheart," Sam said as he tried to comfort his bride.

Sam was heartbroken to hear he couldn't ride to the hospital in the ambulance with Eva. He held his chest, feeling the deep pain inside his heart, as they lifted Eva into the ambulance. "I love you, sweetheart. Till we meet again," Sam called out. Eva blew him a kiss as the ambulance doors closed.

Remaining at the party only long enough to thank everyone for their love and support, Sam hurried to the hospital. Eva had been transferred to the Coronary Care Unit. The emergency room physician was concerned with Eva's irregular heart rhythm and felt she needed careful monitoring before hip surgery the next afternoon. All of this was explained to Sam before he entered Eva's room. "Oh, how small she looked in that bed," thought Sam. Her beautiful party dress had been replaced with a standard, drab hospital gown. IVs were in both arms, and she was receiving oxygen. The metal poles and rope pulleys needed for traction had overtaken her bed. He so desperately wanted to take her place, to save her the pain and anguish she was feeling. The sad pain he felt in his heart was nothing compared to what she was going through.

Eva opened her eyes and smiled at Sam. As usual, her first concern was not for herself but for Sam. "Sit down, sweetheart. You have to be exhausted." Sam replied, "Hush there, I'm fine," as he slid quietly into the chair next to her bed. He reached for her hand and gently caressed it until Eva was once again asleep. It took a lot of convincing to get Sam to go home for the night. He felt comfortable enough to leave only after he was given the direct number to the unit and the nurse's solemn promise to call him if Eva needed him. The tears in his eyes validated his sadness at having to spend their first night apart in their 63 years together. Sam said he would be back early in the morning. "I haven't missed a single morning of saying 'I love you' to my Eva and I'm not about to start now," he shared with the staff.

Eva had a very restless night being away from Sam. She hoped he was having more luck getting to sleep but guessed he probably felt the same way she did. It was nearly dawn before exhaustion took over and Eva fell into a sound sleep. True to his word, Sam was at the hospital before 7:00 AM. The night nurse updated him on Eva's condition and introduced me as the day nurse just coming on duty. She told Sam that she and Eva had talked off and on for most of the night because Eva just couldn't sleep without him. "I know how she feels. My heart was aching so much for her. But, I'm here now and need to start our day by telling her I love her. Can I see her?" "Sure," I said, "but don't wake her if she's still asleep." "I promise," Sam said as he walked toward her room.

After report, I stood up to follow the night nurse into Eva's room for bedside rounds. Briefly delayed by another coworker, I was startled to hear, "I need help!" As I turned toward Eva's room, I saw Sam falling forward as the night nurse struggled to hold him upright. His head struck the traction apparatus as he pitched forward and crumpled to the floor. It was only because Eva was so totally exhausted that she miraculously slept through the commotion at the foot of her bed.

We carefully pulled Sam out into the hallway and closed Eva's door. We had no alternative but to attempt resuscitation right outside her room. For 20 minutes, we did everything we could to save Sam. The hallway was littered with paraphernalia from the code. Several of us cried as the cardiologist called an end to the code. I had spent the last 20 minutes kneeling at Sam's side trying to give him the benefit of my 16 years of CCU experience.

As I started to get up, I was flabbergasted when Sam took a deep breath and opened his eyes. It took me a few seconds to comprehend what my eyes were seeing! I barely whispered, "Sam, are you awake?" Words left me as Sam turned toward me and nodded his answer to my question. It is very difficult to describe the feelings of exhilaration and amazement that rushed through each of us as we placed Sam back on the monitor and gently moved him onto a stretcher.

Sam's EKG showed a complete heart block, and as we wheeled him into the procedure room, we explained to him the need for a temporary pacemaker. He was able to give written consent, astonishing us all. The pacer went in without any problems, and within 15 minutes, Sam's vital signs had completely stabilized without any residual from his earlier cardiac arrest.

Sam motioned to us that he wanted the endotracheal tube out, and because his condition was very stable, the cardiologist agreed. It hadn't even been an hour since Sam's heart had stopped and he was now asking us where he was, what had happened, and how Eva was. After we told Sam about the entire ordeal, Sam smiled at us with a "Thank you. I need to say 'Good Morning' to my bride. Please get her on the phone for me." He was adamant, ignoring our pleas that he needed to rest right now.

The night nurse who was by now physically and emotionally exhausted, went back into the unit to find Eva awake. She called into the procedure room and I helped Sam hold the receiver. His face brightened as he heard Eva's gentle voice. Sam responded, "Good morning, sweetheart. I love you very much," to which Eva replied, "I love you too, Sam." Promising Eva that he was in no pain and that he would see her shortly, he whispered, "Till we meet again" into the phone.

I had just hung up the phone when the monitor alarm went off. When I turned around, I was devastated to see that Sam's heart had once again stopped. Despite a full resuscitative attempt, we were unable to restart Sam's heart. He was pronounced dead at 0825, nearly an hour and a half after his first arrest.

Having to face Eva was perhaps one of the hardest things I have ever had to do as a nurse. Eva thanked the cardiologist for all that he had done. She remained so calm and collected that I feared she hadn't truly understood what had been told to her. As we turned to leave the room, she held my arm and asked me to stay for a minute. I sat on the edge of her bed as she smiled at me. "Are you wondering why I'm not crying?" she asked. I shook my head, fearful of saying the wrong thing. She explained, "He couldn't go until he had wished me good morning and to say he loved me. Sam always keeps his promises." Sam's last words, "Till we meet again" echoed in my thoughts as Eva fell back asleep. It was then that I realized just how small she did look in that hospital bed.

Anxious to Leave

Rumona Dickson

I worked as a specialty area float nurse and was sent to the Coronary Care unit. I had frequently been assigned there, and knew most of the staff well. This night, my assignment was a woman who had experienced a fairly serious heart attack (myocardial infarction). She had been in the unit for almost a week. The staff was very fond of her, and because of that, they usually did not allow an "outsider" to care for her. When I arrived in the unit, I was told she was experiencing heart failure, and because all the nurses were so close to her, they did not feel they could care for her in case of a cardiac arrest.

I entered her room to find her sleeping. Her heart rate was slow and her blood pressure was being maintained solely by two different intravenous drugs. In spite of continuous oxygen, her skin was gray, cool, and damp to the touch. As I always do, even with comatose patients, I introduced myself by name and said I would be her nurse for the evening. It was then I received my first shock. Even though she appeared to be unconscious, she opened her eyes, greeted me in a most polite manner, and told me how pleased she was to meet me.

Closing her eyes, she appeared to sleep while I did my initial assessments. She drifted in and out of consciousness, and on several occasions, woke with a start and with a disappointed look on her face. At one point, she told me she preferred not to wake up there again, giving me the impression she had been someplace else! My patient did, however, ask to see her son. He had been called to the bedside, but did not come because he was not able to watch his mother die.

That evening, her own doctor came to see her. He was a close friend as well as her physician. She told him she was very pleased he had been able to come and say, "Goodbye," and that she hoped he would tell her son that she understood why he had not come. Her doctor denied to her that she was dying and left the room without even holding her hand.

She commented to me, "He's my age, and it must be very hard for him to see me going to such a beautiful place when he has to stay here."

I spoke with her doctor who reiterated that his patient was not going to die and that we must do everything we could to help her survive. In the days before the popularity of "Do Not Resuscitate" orders, we did all we could to revive patients, even though sometimes we knew they might not want to be revived. Even though my contact with this patient had been limited, I knew that I would be unable to call a code in the event of a cardiac arrest, so I went to the nurses at the central cardiac monitoring system and told them I was turning off the monitor in the room. In case her heart stopped, they could call the code and perform the resuscitation. But I knew that they would not.

When I returned to her room, she again awoke abruptly and said, "Oh, damn." She quickly apologised and told me she had never sworn out loud in her life, and I believed her. Then she began telling me where she had been when her eyes were closed. She told me of the brilliant colours, the wonderful feelings of peace, and the presence of beautiful angels. Wanting to stay there, she was disappointed with each awakening. Even though she thought I was a wonderful person, she was really anxious to cross over to this other world.

She asked me if I was religious and asked me to pray with her. We said The Lord's Prayer together and then she requested the 23rd Psalm. We recited it together, and at this point, the tears were quietly streaming down my cheeks. She reached up and wiped away the tear from my cheek, thanked me so much for being there, and closed her eyes for the final time.

At that moment, one of the nurses who had been at the central monitor came into the room to check on my patient and me. She wanted to make sure everything was all right, since the central monitor had revealed that my patient's heart had not shown any activity for several minutes.

Had I been the one to see an angel too?

Unfinished Business

Pat Obenour

My hospice patient was a woman with a strong and active religious faith who was very open about her beliefs. Her children had returned home to be with their mother in her last days. One day when I went for our visit, she told me she knew she was going to heaven very soon—that the angels had come to see her. Flushed with joy, she told of how they had filled the room and touched her arm lightly, creating a very pleasant tickling sensation. Her daughters validated that indeed, something had happened that night, as they heard their mother laughing, giggling, and talking in a voice stronger and clearer than she spoke during the day. When I asked for a description of the angels, she said they all had blonde hair and wore robes of a soft, beautiful peach color.

My patient told me she could hardly wait to die, to be with the angels! Every morning that she woke up still in her own bed, she felt disappointed. Several weeks earlier when we first began visiting her, she expressed a strong belief that she was going to be miraculously cured, but shortly thereafter, she said she had been told by Jesus that she had unfinished business to complete. The next week, she shared with me that the business was finished and she was ready to go.

She had such a beautiful faith that radiated from her to others until the day she died. Her family was supportive and loving, and I felt very privileged to have been invited in at such an intimate time of their lives.

It's Time to Release Him

Cindy

It was a slow night in our normally busy surgical intensive care unit. However, when the trauma pager went off, we knew our slow night was about to pick up. The call was a sad one. Coming to us from the emergency room was a 40-year-old gentleman with a history of bipolar disorder who had shot himself in the head in a suicide attempt. It was a bad wound, and his prognosis was poor.

His mother accompanied him to the unit, and knowing that his days could only be a few, I chose to allow her to come and go at will, a forbidden act in this unit. Throughout the night, he made no respiratory effort of his own, his chest rising and falling with the steady hiss of the ventilator. At no time did he open his eyes, move any muscle, or show any signs of recovery. His heart rate remained regular and rhythmic, but it was obvious that only the barest of brainstem function was left.

His mother would come in, hold his hand, and whisper in her son's ear. She told us loving stories of her son as a child, before the terrible specter of mental illness appeared, eventually leading him to this fate. She rarely left the unit, desiring to stay by his side instead. At three in the morning, she asked me what, in my experience, I felt was the length of time he could remain alive on life support, and I replied that only God knew. I shared with her that I believed it was important for her to talk to her son and share thoughts with him so he would not feel so alone. She looked at me in the dim lights of the nighttime unit and said through the shadows, "I know the angels are with him now. It is time to release him from his torment in this world." And with that, she walked to his bedside and whispered in his ear. She kissed him, smiled at me, and walked out the door.

I sat by his bedside, and at 3:07 AM, just minutes after his mother left, his heart suddenly fluttered and within seconds, stopped. His swollen eyes strained open and looked skyward. As he lifted his

52

seemingly lifeless arms toward heaven, he died peacefully. In that seven-minute span of time, I was convinced he gave himself up to the angels, dying as his mother had whispered in his ear, "Go to the angels, son. They are here to free you."

Nina's Angel

Irene Jones

Nina was my grandmother. She and I were very close, so close that we shared the same middle name, Irene. When Nina's health began to deteriorate, I started thinking about the shortage of health care personnel in America. Nina loved to tell me what an angel I was and that I should become a nurse because I was so compassionate and caring. Nursing was always my dream, but because I was a young mother with two small children, it was not a financial option at the time.

Nina died one day in 1984, two floors below, where I was hospitalized for Rocky Mountain Spotted Fever. I was not able to be with her because I was too sick, but the night she died, I was jolted awake by her voice. I dreamed that she had died but that she would not allow the nurses to turn off the lights or pull the sheet over her head because her work was not yet finished. She had not yet talked to me.

Later, my mother told me Nina had asked to see me the night she died, but she understood why I was unable to be there. Filled with grief for weeks, I told my husband I had to follow my heart and go to nursing school.

Summer was nearing its end, and I was third on the waiting list. It looked like I would have to wait another year to live my dream. But in August, on my birthday, the phone rang. The school called to tell me the two people ahead of me had withdrawn their applications. So, in September of the next year, I graduated with a Diploma in Practical Nursing. I took my state boards in October, on Nina's birthday.

My first job after receiving my license was a private duty case for Georgia, named after the state where she was born. She had lost her husband several months previous, and was experiencing some depression over his death. Because she received kidney dialysis treatments that left her very weak, I went with her to her appointments. I prepared her meals and medications, and took her shopping. This was like being with Nina again! I loved it!

I know Nina was with me through this time, and I suspect she had probably gotten together with Georgia's husband up there also, as his name was Dale, like mine. But wait! There are more coincidences! Dale's sister was the one who hired me and she had the same middle name as my grandmother and me.

Dale's sister was a registered nurse who I would later discover took care of Nina on the night she passed away. Yes, she remembered my grandmother very well, and she shared with me what Nina had said to her about me—that I was her angel, that she wished I could be there with her that night, and that she loved me very much. And that someday God would send her an angel to take care of their family just like the one she had.

This was my final message from Nina. I was the nurse I was meant to be!

This Death

Patricia Taylor

Nothing had prepared me for this death. I have been a nurse for twenty years, most of the time spent working with critically ill and dying patients. I have sat at countless bedsides, holding hands and supporting family members of the dying. I have said many times, "She is gone." The waiting was often difficult. Death may have the final say, but people usually fight that last breath with their whole being. And I can be so patient, so brave, so controlled...at a stranger's death.

But this death was my mother's. She was lying in the bed, unconscious, with shallow, irregular breathing and purple-cold hands and feet. For the last nine months, I had dreaded this night—this night when the colon cancer that had invaded her abdomen finally grew strong enough to steal her life. I had prayed earnestly that I would be there when the end came. And, here I was, alone with my dying mother in the middle of the night. But where were my patience, my bravery, and my control now? I longed for her to talk to me—there were at least a hundred things I needed to ask her. I needed her to comfort me—she was always the one who took care of me. I wanted her to live to the age of 100—but she was only 63.

Actually, the last few weeks had been what I thought were some of her happiest. The family had supported her decision to stop chemotherapy and to refrain from forcing herself to eat. So, with the help of a wonderful hospice nurse, she had four glorious weeks at home without pain, nausea, and diarrhea—30 days filled with loving care from family and friends.

She clapped with child-like delight when the family gathered to blow out candles on the birthday cake she was too ill to eat. Talking into a tape recorder for hours, she stored happy, priceless memories we will forever treasure. Old photo albums were brought out of storage so that long forgotten relatives could be identified. She wrote letters to each of her five children, to be read after she was gone. Remembering her mother who she lost as a teenager, she looked forward to a reunion. And, finally, she talked about her constant faith in a loving God.

So, this heartbreaking night, I played Handel's "Messiah" on the CD and pulled the wicker couch where I lay next to her bed. Placing my head on her pillow with my hands on her arm, I told her how much I would miss her. I smiled when I remembered her last words to me. Asking if she knew who I was, she replied, "Yes, you're the nurse."

Dozing off and on, I would awake with a start and check her breathing to see if it was still there. The coolness in her hands was moving slowly to her shoulders, and I knew that death was creeping up on us.

Mother came to me in a happy, peace-filled dream that intertwined with silent sleep. She was healthy and running barefooted over a grassy field toward a woman with outstretched arms that I at first thought was me. I looked again—it was her mother she was running to. I laughed with joy, and wanted to run alongside my mother, but was prevented from doing so. I couldn't move. She must go without me.

Waking suddenly to an Alleluia chorus, I felt great joy, and then I realized my mother's body was dead. But, the dream upheld me and I knew where her spirit was. I lay for a long time, holding my mother and feeling very peaceful, until the sun's rays rushed in to fill dawn's shadows.

The peace I felt did not last. Family, friends, pastors, nurses, and funeral directors filled the house. Mother's body was wheeled out on a gurney with a cover over her just like all other dead bodies, never to be seen again but turned to ash. Peace turned to numbness, and then to raw, unrelieved pain that lasted an eternity. I will always cherish that night. It was a time of great mystery and wonderful intimacy that I shared with my beloved mother, just like the closeness she shared with me at my birth, and my grandmother with her years before that.

The Light

Naomi Follis

It was a typical cold, dreary winter morning in Northwest Indiana, as my friend and colleague, Billye, and I walked onto the third floor to make our rounds. Just four months from finishing nursing school, and looking forward to our weekend off, we were full of excitement and anticipation. However, nothing we had learned before had prepared us for what we would encounter this day.

Room 305 was our first stop. The chart identified the patient as: Smith, E., 85, widow, black, female, mastectomy—radical with metastasis. Prognosis: terminal.

We had taken care of Mrs. Smith for the past week, so we knew her as a quiet, cooperative woman who enjoyed her son's visits and never complained. Aware of her diagnosis, she chose quiet acceptance. Life was a daily process, for the most part routine, except for today.

Intent on our "to do" list, we entered the room ready to give Mrs. Smith a cheery good morning, when suddenly we stopped. The lights were off in the room, yet the area by the window where Mrs. Smith slept was illuminated with a light brighter than the sun. It took a few seconds for us to remember the sun was not shining on this dreary winter morning.

Mrs. Smith was talking to someone. Her blind eyes looked upward to the place beside her bed where he stood. A wondrous peace and beauty shone on her face, as she nodded her head in agreement. We heard her whisper, "Yes, Lord. I know. I know." We stood riveted to the floor, as if an invisible shield held us away from the lighted area. We held on to each other, as tears stung our eyes and rolled down our cheeks.

Then, the light was gone, leaving the room pale in the early morning gloom. We paused briefly, and took a deep breath before approaching her bed. How do you ask a blind woman about the marvelous light around her bed, or about eyes that have seen more than those with vision ever could? Finally, Billye found enough voice to speak, "We thought we heard voices. Was someone here?"

"Yes," she whispered, "The Lord came to visit me this morning." Her reply was sufficient for us—we did not continue our questioning.

On Monday morning, we hurried down the hall to Mrs. Smith's room, only to find it empty. Of course, we knew she had passed away, and searched for someone who could tell us about the event. The nurse in charge simply shook her head and smiled. "Oh no," she said, "Mrs. Smith has been moved to another room. She's going home today." We found our patient sitting up in bed, feeding herself breakfast, and chatting cheerfully with her new roommate.

Billye and I never told anyone about what happened in Mrs. Smith's room that cold, dreary morning, nor have we mentioned it to each other. It seemed unnecessary, since we could not be sure of what our eyes had seen and what our hearts had perceived. There were simply no words to explain it.

Waiting for Her Son

Susan Schultheis

The patient was in his late sixties when a sudden illness necessitated hospitalization and mechanical ventilation. His prognosis was very poor, and the physicians said if he did survive, he would be dependent upon the ventilator for the rest of his life. Family members chorused, "Save Daddy! Life on the ventilator would be okay. Do whatever you must to keep him alive."

The patient's eldest daughter was the leader of the chorus. But, then something happened. After spending the night asleep in our hospital waiting room, she approached her father's hospital bed with a different air. The nurse assigned to her father asked if she was all right, and she asked to talk with the nurse outside the room.

During the night, the daughter dreamed that a woman dressed in old, 20's-style, clothing came to her and told her that she was waiting for her son. She said she was eager to see him and give him a big hug. Then she told the daughter to tell her father that the woman in the dream loved him.

It seems that the patient's mother died when he was about two weeks old and he had never found a picture of her. Additionally, he had not spoken about her in years.

The family elected to withdraw life support and their loved one died within two hours. Was his mother waiting for him? The nursing staff certainly thought so.

A Final Message of Love and Hope

Edith M. Poidomani

I recently lost my father-in-law to inoperable lung cancer. A man who yielded to anything life had to offer, be it good or bad, he accepted his cancer and lived with positive thoughts right up to the day he died. As we weathered this tremendous loss, I reflected back to the time he learned his brother had inoperable lung cancer. During this difficult time, my father-in-law never lost hope for his brother. In fact, he was an enabler of hope and comfort, believing that without hope, life was being abandoned. Unfortunately, his brother was unable to express his emotions about his diagnosis, and became a shell of a man so unlike his jovial and gregarious previous self.

As a nurse, I felt helpless. I wanted to comfort my father-in-law's brother, but at the same time, I was puzzled over a recurring dream about an elderly woman whom I had never met. In the dream, however, I knew she was the deceased mother of my father-in-law and his brother. Her message was clear and insistent, "Tell him I'm here and I love him and everything is going to be o.k."

I believe that dreams can be inspirational and healing and that they can be part of a learning process of the teacher or messenger. My dilemma: ignore the dream or try to do something positive with it. Should I share it with my father-in-law's brother? Unsure of how he would receive the information, I debated for days before deciding to go ahead and tell him about the dream.

With great trepidation, I entered his hospital room, not knowing that my father-in-law was standing in the far corner. With cracking voice and holding back tears, I explained to him why I was there. After receiving the message, he took my hand, knelt at the foot of the bed, turned his eyes upward to the ceiling, and said, "Thank you, Momma. Now I can die." I will never forget that peaceful moment or my father-in-law's pale and sad face as he quietly left the room with bowed head.

That night, as I drove home from the hospital, I was flushed with warmth in my heart, knowing I had made the right decision. He died shortly after that visit.

Through subsequent discussions with my father-in-law, I knew he was moved by this event. As he contemplated his own imminent death, I hoped he had found some solace from the dream. My father-in-law's cancer was emotionally and physically exhausting to him. During the final stages of his illness, his thoughts and feelings were not always concrete. He left this world as quietly as he lived.

After his death, I could not forget what a good father and husband he had been. A person that loved life, he especially enjoyed working and being outdoors. I believe there is meaning and purpose to one's existence, and that although the body dies, the spirit lives on. My father-in-law's loyalty to his family will remain forever spiritual. And, I know his mother and his brother were there with him giving him that final message of love and hope.

My Angel Has Come Back

Rumona Dickson

Sometimes when working with a patient, I use therapeutic touch, a technique of passing energy from one person to another. When I use this technique, I do not pray for recovery or for healing. I simply use my hands to pass energy, believing it is for the recipient to use in the way they choose.

I had an opportunity to use therapeutic touch on an elderly woman in my care. She had serious heart problems, and when she called for me, I found her pulse to be very irregular and fast, and her blood pressure was 80 over 0 (this was not a good sign). She said she felt weak and short of breath, but in no pain. We called her cardiologist who ordered some medications. As we waited for them to take effect, I remained with my sleeping patient as she slept, practicing therapeutic touch for several hours. When the monitors showed her heart was beating normally, I left for the day.

Two days later, I returned for the evening shift. As I was making my evening rounds, I entered this same patient's room. I had not spoken yet when I entered the room and she was facing the windows, away from me. As I entered the doorway, she immediately stopped talking, did not turn around, and said to her friend, "My angel has come back." She then turned around and greeted me with the most wonderful smile!

She explained that she could feel my energy when I entered the room and then she relayed to us the feeling of calm that she felt on the night she had been so ill. She said she did not need to see me with her eyes to know who was at the door.

This experience was very moving for me.

Divine Intervention

Denise Page-DeMorst

A couple of weeks after my grandmother passed on following a very painful struggle with pancreatic cancer, I was overcome with the terrible, wrenching ache of losing her. I was alone in the house and sitting in a chair weeping and feeling a black hopelessness. Then I became aware of a presence, not visible, but nonetheless a presence. A wonderful feeling of warmth poured over my whole body and I then felt rather than heard that my grandmother was O.K.—that she was so much better now where she was. The feeling was incredible! So much love, comfort, and peace were passed into me. Mere words cannot describe what I felt.

It revived my soul and since that time, I have not been afraid of death. Whenever my faith in the Divine starts to dwindle, I use this memory to help refresh my beliefs. Even without asking, God knew what I needed at that time and helped me through it. I feel very blessed to have been visited by this "presence."

Immune Suppressed Unit 1330

George Heath

I bathed a Japanese man today and he died. I actually bathed him several times as the dysentery drained his life out of him. A man about my age. A man that was doing very well in his profession. Like me. A man with sibling and parents. Like me. A man that did not have a wife, like me, because he was gay, but a man with a lover. Like my wife and me.

A man that wanted his gaunt body to remain clean as much as I wanted him clean. This is my third day with him. In the haze of drug and disease, he has remembered a form of my name, Georgysan. "Georgysan! Georgysan! I need help!"

This means that he is soiled again. He has not called for water or food, to be turned, or medication for pain. He wants to be clean. He takes a little of the nourishment I offer. Is pleased that I medicate him without his asking, but he must be clean.

His chart now has a no code order. If he starts to die, I will comfort him. "Georgysan! Georgysan!" I hear all the way out to the hall, where usually his voice barely makes it across his room. I enter, worried. He needs to be cleaned again.

This time, I set him up in a chair after cleaning more than just what was needed. I give his skin lotion for the second time today. I place powder in skin folds. I take trouble to find the freshest sheets. I make crisp corners.

As I turn to lift him up, his eyes stare straight into mine. He asks, "Georgysan, am I clean now?" I respond, "Yes, Mr. Yamamoto, you are clean enough to receive the emperor." A smile, the first smile I have seen from him, appears on his face. The smile fades. He asks with curiosity, "Georgysan, why is it so dark?" I realize that he is suffering from a low blood pressure, so low that blood is not reaching his retina. That is why it is dark. I cannot feel a radial pulse.

The instinct to lift him up in the bed to get blood circulating, as it should, rises in me. He will be dead in minutes if I don't. Some force other than my trained responses holds me back. I lie. "It is a cloud passing over," I say, looking out the window at a rare, perfectly blue, LA sky. "It looks like the Buddha. Why don't you rest one moment and then I will return you to your bed?" "Yes," he responds, "I am clean. I will rest a moment and think of the Buddha." He bows his head. In less than a couple of minutes, his breathing, and then his pulse, stops.

I did not know it then, but to enter death in a clean state was very important for this Japanese man of a particular Buddhist sect. I know that many of my Christian brethren would condemn me for letting him think of Buddha at the end. There was something stronger than any training or belief could dictate what to do.

In one moment, as Florence Nightingale wrote in her book, *Nurses Notes*, I was able to put myself in the patient's place, more so than any other patient. For one extremely thin slice of time, I felt his experience and knew what he wanted.

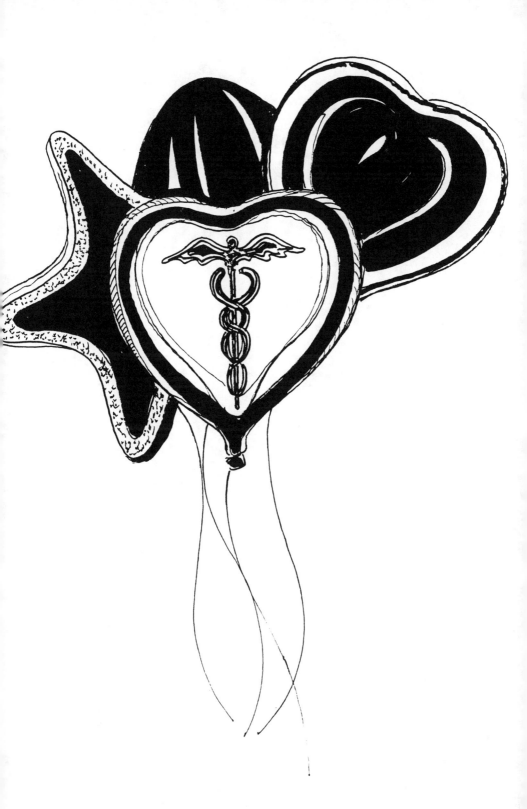

3

The Essence of Care Giving: Serving with Love

Nurses enter nursing for many reasons—to learn and practice within the field of health care, to show our empathy for others, to be around people, to help the sick get well, to make enough money to support ourselves and our families, to grow personally, and many others. The reasons are too numerous to count.

Now nurses will share with you our deepest, heartfelt feelings about why we decided on this sometimes difficult career when so many other possibilities, sometimes more financially rewarding, were beckoning to us. Come with us as we journey to and through the heart, the essence, of nursing.

Just to Be There

Louise M. Nelson

When I worked as a private duty nurse, I cared for a woman who had undergone a mastectomy. Before the surgery, she was told the lump would be identified and biopsied, and if found to be cancerous, the tumor, along with the breast, would have to be removed. Unfortunately, that is what had to be done, and when the surgeon came the next morning to tell the patient the outcome of the operation, she said, "I know." She had figured it out from the bulky dressing on her chest. On the whole, the patient was grateful to have received an early diagnosis, and felt optimistic about her recovery. Also, she had a very supportive family who was there to help her through this difficult time.

Two days after surgery, when it was time for the first dressing change, she asked me, rather anxiously, to stay with her. I held her hand, feeling totally useless. As the surgeon removed the bulky dressing that had served as a camouflage, my patient began to cry at the first sight of her mutilated chest. I could say nothing as I stayed by her side and felt some of her pain.

When the procedure was over and her tears were dried, this patient turned to me and thanked me with deep gratitude for helping her! All I had done was stand there holding her hand, not saying a word, yet this woman felt my sympathy and caring. I learned then that sometimes nothing can be done. You just have to be there and care.

The Haitian Baby

Paula Schneider

"What should we do for this little one?" I asked Dr. Seay with desperation. She turned, looked at me with her clinical eyes full of compassion. Our little patient was obviously very ill, too malnourished to take a deep breath, and ready to give up. We had seen many children over the past three days at our makeshift clinic in Petit Guave, Haiti, but this one was clearly the sickest.

"Well, first we should give him a gentle bath, and try to give him some diluted baby formula. After you do those two things, bring him back to me," she replied. My husband, Larry, and I quickly set up a basin for washing. As we removed the dirty tea towel the baby was wrapped in, I looked into the mother's very worried face. She knew things were not going well and that her baby was very ill. She, herself, was very thin and emaciated. We gloved and began to gently wash our young patient. He was too ill to do anything but emit a whimper that remains forever etched in my memory. His pain was more than any of us could bear. As we trickled the water over his broken skin that was peeling away from his body, I cried.

Larry and I both cried, and spoke to the baby softly as we did so. Time stood still for us as we ministered to our little patient the best we could. I felt at once outraged and sad to think of the poverty in this little country only a short distance from the mainland of America. Most Americans don't understand the poverty there—they hear it, they might even see pictures of it, but until you have seen it with your own eyes, you don't know it. How could we, who have so much, allow this type of suffering in an innocent baby?

The bathing ended. We had done all we could. We patted his little body dry and handed him back to his mother in a clean sheet. He was too tired, exhausted, and ill to even cry. The silence roared around us. I handed the mother a baby bottle with some diluted formula in it, and through an interpreter, explained to the mother how to attempt to feed her baby. She seemed to understand, and she disappeared into the sea of dark faces.

Nobody was smiling.

Shortly, someone from the crowd rushed to us. Our little patient had died in his mother's arms, too long without nourishment to be able to take it now. Everything in the busy clinic came to a halt for a few minutes as we each reflected on what this event meant in our lives, our busy lives, our thing-filled lives. Each of us on the medical team was sad, but we had more patients to see that day. All total, we saw over 850 patients in the three days we were there.

So, as a nurse, what did this mean to me? My personal belief is that we call forth our own life experiences in order to learn, grow, and remember who we are and why we are here. So how was I to respond to this incredibly sad event? I gave thanks for this experience, then and now. I felt grateful to have been able to ease the little one's pain, if only for a few minutes, with the cool, fresh water that cleaned his little body. That, to me, is what nursing is all about—having the opportunity to ease someone else's pain, if only for a short while.

Nursing is Unique

Peter Ramme

At any given time, somewhere on our planet, there is a nurse who is present, awake, alert, and attentive to the immediate health needs of one or more people. All day, all night, every day, and every night—many of us are actively practicing our professions.

Nurses work within intimate range of vulnerable people at crucial times in their lives. We often take over vital physiologic functions, emotional roles, basic physical care, and timely responses to skillfully determined needs. We are the only professionals who practice physiology with humans, carrying knowledge about how to do this that is written in our expertise developed through a complex integration of skills, learning, and an ever-growing base of knowledge. Alert nurses learn something new and unique about human beings practically every day.

Nurses are consistently among the most trusted of professionals. Patients trust us to administer complex care in an expert fashion and we are believed because we are accustomed to being truthful and accurate in our communications. People know that our work is arduous, and they usually deeply appreciate what we do.

We are responsible for knowing and respecting individuals within their lives, lifestyles, cultures, beliefs, hopes, and expectations of care. We work in the arena of human relationships and draw our knowledge from sciences, arts, religions, and many other disciplines. This awareness is applied daily to help patients on their unique paths toward health and wholeness.

Nursing is a performing art, a contact sport, a life's calling, and a cascade of deeply spiritual human rewards. Many people live their entire life without many kinds of care. Virtually no one goes through life without needing some kind of nursing care.

We share the entire range of critical human experiences—from birth to death—with other people who have no other bond to us than the nurse-patient relationship. We understand such experiences because we live through them with so many people in the course of our practices. We see and share these experiences from a vantage, and in a depth and breadth that no other profession can. Nursing is an integrated, living practice that requires us to possess all the qualities, skills, and experiences mentioned here, and more.

We are typically quiet about what we do and the knowledge we possess. We hold the keys to health care of the future. We have the knowledge to carry health care forward when the current spasm of greed-oriented corporate fascism is a distant memory. We have already made key changes and adaptations to assure our profession will continue.

The Caring Lesson

Steve Anderson

One of my first nursing instructors was what you might call old guard. She was rumored to keep a quarter in her pocket to bounce on the patient's bed to make sure the sheets were tight enough. Having worked in hospitals for the past 10 years, I thought I was going to breeze through my first clinical assignment. After all, I felt pretty sure I already knew all there was to know about medicine and nursing. Needless to say, she saw right through me. She knew what I needed, and she gave it to me!

My first patient was a 45-year-old male, otherwise very healthy, who had unfortunately suffered a stroke two days earlier. His condition was stable, he was fairly independent in his care, and did not require a lot of nursing expertise at this point. In fact, he was scheduled to be discharged the next day. I approached my nursing instructor, asking what it was that I was supposed to do for my patient, and she replied, "Just go sit with him and talk with him."

We talked about his life, his family and children, and his true love, the trumpet. As he told me of the way he loved to play this musical instrument, I will never forget the look on his face when he asked, "Will I ever be able to play again?" I mumbled something like, "I don't know," but when I looked up, I could see by the tears in his eyes that he already knew the answer. I began to cry too. I reached out to grab his hand, and we sat there—two grown men—holding each other's hands and blubbering like babies. At some point, my instructor walked into the room, smiled, said nothing, and left us alone.

At our evening conference to discuss our patients and the day's events, she said nothing about what she had seen in my patient's room. I stayed late that day to ask what those few touching moments with my patient meant and how she knew it would happen that way. She smiled and told me, "You were ready for this lesson," the lesson of caring. That, to me, is what nursing is all about.

Thank you, Betty Witt. And may God bless all the Betty Witts out there who are providing us the opportunity to learn the lessons we are ready for.

Hope

Rosemary Meganck

Some days you get up and go to work and you find yourself wondering why you became a nurse. You wonder, "Am I doing any good at all or am I just beating my head against a wall?" On other days, it is like waking up from a daydream and getting slapped in the face. "This is why you became a nurse, you dummy!"

I recently had one of those days. I've been a nurse for nearly 20 years, first working in labor and delivery and more recently as a certified nurse midwife. As a midwife, I am primarily responsible for my own caseload, but I work closely with obstetricians. We ask them for advice on more complicated patients and they look to us for advice on alternative childbirth approaches. Sometimes we even manage patients together.

A few months ago, one of my physician colleagues approached me about a patient of his who was HIV positive and would soon be delivering her second child. She had been infected with the virus that causes AIDS by a previous partner, but only discovered that she was HIV positive after her second marriage, when her pregnancy was diagnosed.

Instead of falling apart, this amazing couple gathered their emotional and spiritual reserves and got on with the business of adding a baby to their family. Mrs. C. took very good care of her health and took AZT to minimize the risk of transmitting the virus to her unborn baby. Her husband and first child tested negative for the virus.

Mrs. C. had a natural birth attended by a midwife with her first child. She had breastfed her son and assumed she would be able to do so again with the second child. Unfortunately, she would not be able to this time. When her physician told me about her and asked if I could provide teaching and support, I agreed to meet with her and her husband.

We spent about an hour in my office, talking about the upcoming birth and their plans for the baby. Her husband wanted to be very involved and to be her primary support. This was his first child, and he was willing and

75

excited to be there for his wife. We talked at length about breastfeeding, something she really treasured with her first child. However, it was not to be.

Call it luck or coincidence if you will, but Mrs. C. went into labor early one morning while I was on duty! Her physician and I agreed to attend the birth together. He would do most of the hands-on and I would be there for emotional support. Her labor proceeded normally, with her husband acting as coach and her mother-in-law as support person.

As she approached the second stage of labor, the excitement in the room quadrupled. The love waiting to greet this little one was vibrating. Her husband could hardly contain his excitement! We did not know if this was to be a boy or a girl, but Mr. C. said he had always wanted a daughter. Grandma was manning the video camera, the nurse was helping Mrs. C. into a more comfortable position, the physician and I were gowned and ready to "catch," and Mrs. C. was as serene as I have ever seen a woman about to give birth.

A perfectly healthy, 8 pound, 3 ounce baby girl was gently pushed into the waiting hands of the physician, and together we lifted a crying baby ever so softly into her mother's outstretched arms, where she immediately quieted. My voice was quivering when I looked at Mrs. C. and asked what she planned to name her new daughter. She looked me in the eye and announced "Hope." I could no longer hold back my tears. I looked around the room in hopes of regaining my composure, but there was not a dry eye in the room. "Tears of hope," I thought.

Mr. and Mrs. C. thanked me for my help, but it is I who must thank them. Every time I am present for a birth, I feel privileged to be allowed to share such an intimate and beautiful moment. This birth gave more to me than I ever could have given. Hope's birth reminded me why I chose the profession I did. She renewed my faith in birth, in motherhood, and in the future. She gave me hope.

A Twist of Fate

Ludovina Archeval

As I set out to make a routine home visit to admit my new patient to the agency for home care services, I never dreamed that the encounter would turn out to be such an uplifting experience! The patient I was assigned to visit was an 82-year-old single female who had just been discharged from the hospital after a one-week stay. She had fallen at home, sustaining a muscle sprain and the week spent in the bed recuperating caused generalized muscle weakness.

So, I made a call to my patient's home, introduced myself, and set up a time for the visit. She told me her niece lived next door and would be there to greet me.

When I arrived at my patient's apartment, she let me in and said her niece and her brother would be there shortly. I proceeded with the admission process, and as we were talking, her brother walked in. "Ludovina, this is my brother, Dr. James Landon," she said as an introduction. As I looked at him, memories of my student nursing days swept over me.

Twenty-nine years earlier, Dr. Landon had been a prominent surgeon who performed many surgeries in the hospital where I attended nursing school. How well I remembered our first encounter!

I was a bundle of nerves as I scrubbed, gowned, and gloved in order to assist the surgeon, and I mentally rehearsed how I would pass the instruments, sutures, and dressings during surgery. However, Dr. Landon grumbled when he realized a student nurse would assist him, and this made me even more uncomfortable.

His displeasure with having a student nurse in the operating room made me increasingly apprehensive, and my mind went totally blank as I tried to remember what I was supposed to do. I looked toward my instructor for guidance, but she was also intimidated and did not offer much support. I managed to make it through the surgery, all the while wishing I had chosen another profession.

That first encounter with Dr. Landon made me uneasy every time I had to assist him on the unit with a dressing change or suture removal. He always barked at the student nurses, and I tried to hide when I saw him coming. In his presence, I always felt inferior.

Now, here we were, together again after 29 years. Fate would have me performing a complete physical assessment on his loved one and discussing with him and his sister the services I, along with other health team members, could provide for her. Today, I was in full control as I skillfully assessed her physical, psychological, and emotional needs, safety factors, and environment. I reviewed her medications and diet, and discussed how frequently nursing visits would be needed as well as home health aide services, physical therapy, and community resources.

Dr. Landon, who obviously did not remember me and our earlier encounters, listened carefully. At the completion of my visit, he told me he was very impressed with my professional manner and with the variety of services his sister would be receiving. At first, he seemed uncomfortable asking me questions about home care, but I patiently discussed the plan of care, and included his sister in the discussion.

Just then, his daughter, my patient's niece, walked into the apartment, apologizing for arriving late. Dr. Landon smiled, saying, "This nurse is very competent, and she has everything under control," to which his daughter replied to me, "I'm only a practical nurse, not a registered nurse like you." I suspected she had been put down for being "only a practical nurse," just as I had been criticized for being "only a student nurse." I responded, "You are a nurse and you have skills and knowledge which you use in your practice. Don't let anyone put you down, and be proud of what you know and what you can do to help others."

As I left, Dr. Landon's daughter gave me a big smile and said she really looked forward to our next visit. My patient thanked me for coming, and Dr. Landon shook my hand and said he would probably see me again on the next visit also.

I felt uplifted and full of pride. I realized that my knowledge and skills in nursing had prepared me well to overcome the inferiority I had felt so long ago in the presence of this once overbearing prominent surgeon. I am a nurse, complete with skills, abilities, and knowledge that allow me to help my fellow human beings. Nobody can take that away from me.

Nursing: My Commitment and Reward

Terry L. Steptoe

The American Nurses Association's definition of nursing is *"the diagnosis and treatment of human responses to actual or potential problems."* The profession of nursing has been very good to me. It has provided me with a comfortable salary for the past 16 years. But the definition given above does not begin to completely explain what nursing really is and what it means to me.

The medical business is changing by leaps and bounds these days, but the true mechanics of nursing should never change! Nursing is just what the word says it is. It's coming through a door, leaving your personal problems and feelings at home, to care for those who, for the moment, cannot care for themselves for whatever reason. It means smiling when you may not feel like smiling, physical contact with people who might not always meet your standards, and yes, even sometimes giving someone a gentle hug or the touch of a hand to simply say, "I do care."

After all of this giving and caring, not just to patients but also to physicians and other health professionals, our personal wells sometimes become dry. For me, the filling of the well comes when someone I've cared for says, "Thank you" or smiles or when I see a patient get well in spite of all odds. This is a very important part of being and staying a good nurse. We must occasionally have that re-filling so we know we are at the point in life we need to be. Many nurses achieve this in different ways, and no one way is more correct than the other is.

Nursing also means maintaining high professional standards and staying current with new technology and other changes. It means keeping a flexible and open mind to changing times. The winds of change are blowing, and if flexibility is not part of professional thinking, we will snap like dried-up trees. Keeping this level of professionalism creates not only good patient care, but also confidence and trust in our fellow workers, because teamwork is very important.

Teamwork is also another important factor in nursing. For us to be able to do our jobs and create a positive environment for our patients, we must, *WE MUST*, be able to work together in harmony. We must learn to accept one another as we are, and try to channel all our efforts into the care of the one needing attention—the patient. In this profession, we often put ourselves on the back burner and we have to step back and think, "What is the best for the common goal?" the common goal being the health and well being of our patients.

I am very proud God saw fit to call me into this profession. It takes special people to do special jobs, and nursing is a special job. You nurses are special people! Take pride in what you do and who you are, for beyond a shadow of a doubt, you have been called to a higher place.

I Teach

Peggy

The resident physician shakes his head as he leaves the patient's room and comes toward us. He is despondent, and remarks to a nurse standing nearby, charting, "I can't do anything for them. She is dying, and he wants me to do something." The nurse replies, "Yes, there is something you can do. Here." She hands him a washcloth and towel, saying, "Her pain is under control, but the morphine makes her perspire. Go in and wash off her face with a cool washcloth," and he takes off for the room.

We peek into the room. The resident is gently bathing his patient's face. The patient is sleeping peacefully, and the husband is holding her hand and telling the resident how beautiful she was as a young woman.

Shortly, the resident emerges from the room, smiles at the nurse, and says, "Thank you," while walking away a little lighter than he arrived.

Yeah – I teach.

My Job, My Calling

Marlene Shea

The beginning of my nursing career was somewhat out of the ordinary. I did not want to be a nurse since childhood like a lot of nurses. I had only visited a hospital once, having been a patient in the Emergency Room as a child. And, I never knew anyone who was a nurse. While growing up, this was the farthest thing from my mind. So, how did I become a nurse? Let me tell the story.

At the age of 14, I won a one-year scholarship to a girls' college preparatory high school. My grade school friends were attending different schools, so I never really felt that I fit in, but I did manage to make a few good friends. I was very shy.

In the spring of 1958, near the end of my time there, the school had an assembly for the seniors. Nurses came to recruit new nursing students, and I found myself paying close attention to what these nurses had to say. Afterwards, I thought, "I think I would like to be a nurse."

My parents had already enrolled me in a secretarial training course, so I did not plan to attend college. In fact, my father had already made a down payment on the course. I don't remember how I broached the subject of my attending nursing school with my parents. Shy and unassertive, I generally had a difficult time making up my mind. But, I must have found some resources somewhere, because I managed to take a test and apply to the one nursing school in Northern Kentucky, St. Elizabeth Hospital. I passed the test and began training in August of 1958.

While in nursing school, I stayed in a dormitory at the hospital for three years. This was the first time I had been away from home for any length of time. One weekend when I went home to visit, I overheard my father on the phone saying to my grandfather, "Yes, she is in nursing school, but I don't think she will finish the three-year course." I was very angry and hurt. Of course I would finish! His words turned out to be the one thing that kept me in school.

Shortly after I started nursing school, I began dating a young man who I later married. We had been dating about a year when he began asking me to drop out of school because he didn't like my early weekend curfews and he was ready to get married. (In those days, a student could not be married while in nursing school.) Remembering my father's words to my grandfather, I became increasingly determined to complete my training. My boyfriend and I argued many times over this topic for the next two years. I graduated in 1961 and insisted on working at least one year before I would get married.

I loved nursing from the very beginning. At times, it was hard work and there were long hours, but I always felt this was where I was supposed to be. During the 60's, I worked full time for two years and then part time while I raised three young children. In 1970, I returned to nursing and have been working ever since—always at St. Elizabeth Hospital where I received my training.

There have been many changes in nursing over the years. I've watched my small hospital turn into a Medical Center with three separate facilities. Since 1974, my area of concentration has been Psychiatric Nursing, and I have had the privilege of helping create a Partial Hospitalization Program.

Over the years, I have met such wonderful people and have made strong, lasting friendships. To my amazement, I have been a registered nurse for 36 years. To this day, I know this is where I belong. Nursing remains not only my job but also my calling in life. I thank God for multiple blessings and nudges that pushed me onto the right and perfect path for my life.

Diary of a New Nurse

Ng Xiang Lynn

I wonder how I can be solitary
    When everyone's around?
        I don't know if I'm my own self
        Or responding to the crowd.
          Am I trying to act a role
        Or am I real?

...............or maybe I'm just another ant upon the hill....................

        living day by day

doing things I'm supposed to do
saying what I'm expected to say

        living day by day.

Last week I went to visit a patient in the Intensive Care Unit. Her son came in seconds after I did and was leaning against the door just watching me as I held her hand. He eventually entered the room, and we discussed how much worse her condition had become. He asked me if she would pull through. What do I say? I took refuge in a non-committal "She might—it's a 50/50 chance here."

To me, her condition had worsened. The last time I was here, she was about to be extubated. Her eyes were open and she nodded when I asked if she remembered me. I shared with her son how she cried before her surgery, how she kept telling me she was so afraid she would die on the operating table, how she squeezed my hand as the tears fell from her eyes. I reflected on how I wished I could hold her and cry with her, but felt unable to do so because I was her pillar of strength. I told her she would get well soon and

84

go home—that she could "pang sim" (dialect term for don't worry). She told me about her husband who was dependent on her, and what would he do without her? He still had not been told how ill she was.

Now, she is lying in the ICU with a thousand and one intravenous feeding tubes inserted into her body. She still recognized me, however, and responded when I held her hand and said, "Hi." I encouraged her son to talk to her, and I walked out of the ICU.

These days I find myself afraid to call to find out how she is. She may be dead already. How will her husband and son cope? She taught me the value of an available hand, a listening ear. Nurses don't realize how much these things matter when they are in school.

It's hard to let go when you know someone well. When you see them as a mother and a wife. She told me things people normally keep to themselves. People who are ill and frightened are like that—they tend to confide in whoever will listen.

Being fresh out of school, I was shocked by these new thoughts and emotions. Nursing isn't just another profession. It is a life. Where else can I be with people, watch them grow, live, and die? Where else can I be exposed to all the frailties of life, as well as the strengths? Only as a nurse can a person receive the honor of sharing life at this depth. As nurses, we are all experiencing humanity. And we are all richer for it.

I Understand

Julie G. Matthews

Mrs. P. looked into the mirror and straightened her wig. Sitting atop the dresser were the paintings and drawings she was working on. I stood at the door and watched her smile as she began to draw. I thought, "What does she have to smile about? She's barely 40 years old, is beautiful and talented, and dying of leukemia."

That was 1978, and I was a 20-year-old new graduate, green, and Mrs. P. knew it. She knew I was scared of taking care of a dying patient, and was compassionate with me. Taking me under her wing, she made me feel at ease.

After completing an unsuccessful round of chemotherapy, she knew she would not be going home. Aware that precious time together was short, her 12-year-old daughter and husband visited often.

When I came on duty, I was always drawn to her room first. She was interested in the nurses and their everyday lives. One nurse was expecting and went into labor while at work. Mrs. P. was so excited that day, waiting for Jenny to deliver. It appeared she had the rest of her life for enjoyment, when in fact she had only a few short weeks.

"Julie," she would often say, "Tell me about your family. How old is your daughter? What did y'all do yesterday? Did you take her for a walk?" She seemed to have an insatiable desire to know about everyone's activities. We talked about everything, even memories that were painful for her. The bitterest memory of all was that she had tried for years to become pregnant, to no avail. She and her husband then adopted their sweet daughter at birth. Right before this last exacerbation of her leukemia, she was elated to learn she was pregnant. On the waves of euphoria, she was told her leukemia had returned with a vengeance. To receive the chemotherapy that she needed to have a chance at recovery, she would have to sacrifice the fetus. After having the surgery at another hospital, she came to our Catholic hospital to begin this round of chemo.

Over the days, her condition worsened, and she was placed on oxygen and intravenous fluids. Too weak to speak, she was as beautiful as ever the last time I saw her. All I could do was cry. She talked, and I listened. She was aware that her in-laws were afraid they would catch cancer from her and so they would not come to visit. She told me of her love for her family. And she talked of death—the word that I could not, as a young graduate, mention or understand.

"Julie, I am not afraid of dying. I am a Christian and I am not afraid of death. But, I don't want to leave my family. I don't want to leave them!" These words were spoken with such resolution that I knew she would not leave them. Even in death, I knew that she would take a small piece of them with her and leave some of herself behind. I never saw her again after that evening.

Now, it's 20 years later, and I have taken care of many dying patients. But the memory of that first experience blazes as if it were yesterday. Mrs. P. helped me begin an emotional learning experience that continues today. In retrospect, I believe that was one of her last acts of kindness to a shy, insecure young nurse. She knew that I was a caring person, and she wanted to nurture that caring so I could pass the gift on to others.

"I don't want to leave my family," the dying elderly man cries and I understand.

Our Team Leaders, the Elderly

Linda Lovell

What does teamwork mean in the life a helpless, elderly adult—one who depends on the team of nursing caregivers for his or her very livelihood? What does teamwork mean to me?

As a long-term health care worker, I believe it must mean dedication and commitment to the elderly, to human life. When I look down into a tired, wrinkled face, I stand in awe as that tired face turns into a glowing light with the biggest smile you can imagine just because I walked into the room. This is the moment I realize I have done my share to bring life back into the face and soul of a fellow human being.

As I go through my daily round, I observe co-workers going from room to room, bringing the same kind of smiles to tired, broken bodies. I am reminded of the great gift God has given each of us who work as a team and strive for quality care for our patients. This gift is one of caring, of the ability to bring meaning and love to the face of a tired body.

As my shift draws to an end, and still more dedicated team players come on the scene, I again witness even more acts of kindness such as hugs, kisses, and smiles. Team members who demonstrate, by their actions, that they love the elderly have certainly enriched my life!

As each of us complete our shifts and all routine tasks such as bathing and dressing are carried out, I look around and see the acts of love that go so much deeper than everyday tasks. I see teamwork that truly comes from the heart—health care workers who strive every day to fill a void in the heart of an elderly person. No greater gift has God given to man than the ability to love another human being. Our elderly team members teach us each day how to be team players in the game of life.

The only reason any of my fellow team players can bring a smile to a sad face is because of the lessons we have learned from our patients. The elderly have taught us how to give love freely with no strings attached. I am ever so grateful the elderly head up the team at our facility. They are marvelous teachers and givers!

Angels Away at Camp

Sue Downhill

When I was seven, I went away one summer to a camp in the White Mountains of Montpelier, Vermont. While there, I became very ill with amoebic dysentery, and consequently became very dehydrated. The camp nurse decided I needed to be hospitalized so that I could receive intravenous fluids.

I'll never forget the appearance of that large, uninviting, unfamiliar hospital. Inside, the walls were so high, and it seemed dark to me. I was just a little girl and felt very alone and afraid, even though I knew my parents were on the way and would be there in a couple of days. My private room, with a door, which separated me from the hallways, offered little consolation, except for one frequent visitor—my nurse. Memories of that stay in the hospital have grown dim but for the nurse. She was able to make the whole event a little less scary. She not only helped a little girl get well, but she quieted my fears and made that frightening place a little less so.

Thank you, nurse. Even though I do not know your name, I'm so glad you were there for me. You made my life easier and helped heal me. I think that is the reason I do not fear hospitals the way some others do.

A Chance to Touch

Suzannah Damaa

Thump! The sound of something crashing into the door. Not the usual answer to a knock on a patient's door. I slowly open the door, hoping nothing else will come sailing through the air. "Good morning," I say, "My name is Suzannah and I'm going to be your nurse today." "Hi," she gruffly replies. Knowing that she is not thrilled with my presence and probably hoping that I'll just go away, I ask, "How are you feeling today?" No answer. I really want to help this young woman.

Here before me is a young, athletic college student who has just been admitted because of a suspicion of multiple sclerosis, a serious disease of the nervous system that causes muscle weakness. I search my mind, frantically trying to remember all I can about this disease. What I do remember is that it involves alterations in vision and loss of muscle function. How devastating for this beautiful, strong, young woman before me!

"Why me?" I ask. This is too hard and she is too angry. She is not the quiet, compliant patient pretending to herself and to me that everything's going to be o.k. She wants a fight. She is real, expressing true and raw emotions. I feel she needs me, and so I quickly pull myself together and face this with her head on. I won't be afraid. I will fight desperately to give this woman comfort and friendship, if she will let me.

"May I take your vital signs?" Vital signs—an act so simple, yet so important, so filled with meaning. The chance to touch, to touch gently. Through this simple act, to send a message that I care and that I'll be there. I look her in the eye, remembering that she is a person and not a disease. I put the blood pressure cuff around her arm and search my mind for some outside news to share with her. I want to keep her connected and to remind her that the world is still functioning and that she is a part of that. I suspect she feels very alone and isolated, and so I say, "Did you know that today is Ground Hog Day? Did you ever see the movie *Ground Hog Day*?" A long pause, then she laughs and I laugh with her. I've gotten through!

She has seen the movie and thought it was funny. I experience the greatest joy when she laughs. To me, it says I have given her a second, no, a minute of escape. At this moment, she is not a patient, but a friend. Her pain is far away, and she is laughing. We will be able to work together. We'll struggle, cry, scream, and even throw stuffed animals. We will wrestle with the possibility that she may have a serious condition, but every once in a while, we will step back to escape and to laugh.

Circle of Life

Jeff Reichardt

I am tired. I work so hard.

But lately, I have been especially overworked.

My career has many stresses in it that are inescapable.
>When I started it, I knew I would not get rich.
>I knew this career was a difficult one.
>I knew that respect from fellow professionals was hard won.

I knew that this profession had an image problem with the public.
But I felt I could make a difference.
I felt I could have a positive influence on my chosen career.

I was wide-eyed and naïve, I'll admit, but part of me wishes that reality were different.
Part of me wishes that I could take all of the positives I've received and cancel out all the negatives.

As for the positives, I am thankful that I was able to give a life back to an 18-year-old who is just now learning how to live the life of a quadriplegic.

I feel honored to have been asked to share a bedside prayer for a 12-year-old victim of an accidental gunshot wound who will not survive. His family, in their grief, thought to include me, his caregiver, in the process of saying goodbye.

For these experiences, I am grateful.

For the physicians who took the extra time to ask for my thoughts about the care of OUR patient, I am also grateful.

To the families of hundreds of patients who stopped me in the hall to say, "Thanks," I now say, "Thank YOU."

I say this because I am leaving bedside nursing: I am tired of the politics and back-stabbing. I am tired of all kinds of people who bolster their own pitiful egos by debasing someone else's. I am tired of feeling guilty when I turn down my supervisor's request to stay late for yet another emergency (the fifth one this week).

I am tired of not receiving the respect I deserve—from my co-workers especially. They should be keenly aware of what it takes mentally, physically, and emotionally to perform this, my chosen career.

I am tired of hearing about the shortage of nurses. I know I am burned out. It's a shame.
I consider myself to be a good bedside nurse.

I worry about the next trauma victim and the family as well. Who will take the time to address the total family's needs? Who will sit and hold the hands of the parents who have just signed the organ procurement papers for their dying child, in hopes that some good will come from this tragedy? Who will take care of the body of the infant that just died in the intensive care unit?

It won't be me...

I am tired...

I hurt...

I am not alone, but know that doesn't help...

I feel empty inside...

I can no longer do this to my family or myself...

I am leaving what I love, but how can I?

The truth is, I can't. So, you see, I am refreshed. I still work hard!

Lately, I have been eager to work. My career has many stresses in it that are inescapable. When I began, I knew I would not get rich financially. But my rewards have been many, and much more than money can buy.

I knew that this career would be a difficult one. But, I have always enjoyed a challenge. And I knew that respect from my fellow professionals was hard won, but I forgot that respect is a two-way street.

I knew that this profession had an image problem with the public. But, for a long time, I was just as much a part of the problem as the people that I had begun to disdain.

I know now that I have made a difference.

I am no longer wide-eyed and naïve. I am seasoned and a little wiser.

So, to all the patients, the families, the doctors, and my fellow workers, I say, "Thank you." I cannot leave nursing. I need to be there for the next trauma victim and the family. I need to hold the hands of grieving parents. And, yes, I do need to care for the body of the baby that just died.

It's GOT TO BE ME!

I am refreshed…

I am now whole…

I have not been alone…

I am fulfilled…

I owe it all to my wife and children…

They have reminded me that this is what life is all about.

It's about joy, pain, courage, and sorrow. It's about taking care of each other, meeting each other's needs. It's about renewing life and dignifying death. But, most of all, it's about being human. With all our faults, frailties, strengths, weaknesses, hopes, dreams, and our capacities for kindness and compassion.

In the end, we still carry on. Some say it's through God's will, but I don't know. For me, it's because I cannot turn my back on my fellow man.

It's as simple as that.
For, if we turn our backs, we greatly diminish ourselves.

The Lightning Ridge Experience

Barbara Newman

Lightning Ridge is a unique town in Australia, as it is home to the beautiful black opals, a highly valued gemstone. Because of this wonderful natural attraction, the town blossoms from a population of 700 to 7000 in the spring, when people from all over Australia come to mine for opals. Temperatures are extreme here, ranging from 45 degrees Centigrade during the day to a night temperature of 3 degrees Centigrade.

This ideal setting offers a variety of experiences for nurses and nursing students alike. The one Medical officer in the town is kept very busy in his surgery, while one Registered Nurse and an assistant each staff an 8-hour shift in the Primary Health Care Clinic. My students and I were sent to this delightful health care setting to gain first-hand experience with the limitations, benefits, and demands of working in such a remote and isolated area. We assisted with almost everything, including health promotion programs on diet and preventative education for the school children on using hats and sunscreen to prevent heat exhaustion and sunstroke. On an average day, we saw about 45 patients, with problems ranging from splinters in fingers to more serious problems requiring emergency care. It was in such an emergency that Percy, a miner, was brought to us.

As the ambulance arrived, Percy's motionless body lay on the stretcher covered with a mixture of dirt and blood, and he was unable to respond to questions. He was breathing, but a small amount of blood was trickling from his left eye and a fairly consistent flow of blood was coming from his left leg. As we questioned fellow miners, the students cut away his clothing, hoping all the while that the injuries were not so severe as to require a blood transfusion. His co-workers told us Percy was hurt when a log collapsed, cutting a swathe across his body as it hit his head and leg.

Percy remained unconscious for about 30 minutes, at which time he began to awaken. At first confused, he eventually began to recount what had

96

happened for us, and then gave us a wonderful compliment, saying, "Nurses are the salt of the earth. They have saved my life before, and no doubt if you had not been here this time as well, I might have died."

Truthfully, Percy's assessment of the situation is accurate. The little town of Lightning Ridge is over 600 miles from a major health care institution, and it is generally known that if nurses were not staffing the primary health care facility there, there would be an increase in morbidity and mortality amongst the townspeople.

Percy got to ride in the Air Ambulance that day. Because of his multiple traumas, we decided it would be best to airlift him to a tertiary care facility in Sydney. One of my students who accompanied him on the ride told us later that the flight was uneventful, mainly because it was a warm and clear day; however, there have been instances where the plane has been forced to land in paddocks of outback sheep stations.

We were fortunate to have extra help, in the form of off-duty nurses, to care for Percy. In this remote town, nurses who have left for the day return to assist with a major trauma victim. It is this camaraderie that makes nursing duties and responsibilities bearable in a rural setting such as Lightning Ridge. This team spirit of helpfulness is quite different from working in a metropolitan hospital where the value of mutual support is not a highly prized part of everyday life as it is in small rural settlements of Australia.

We felt lucky to have had this experience. Serving in the clinic in Lightning Ridge was an ideal way to learn about primary health care from a variety of itinerant visitors to this little town. And, Percy taught us about the value of teamwork and the importance of saying "Thanks."

We'll Meet Again Some Day

Norma Singer

I once cared for a young man who was quite ill with AIDS. So ill that the first day we met we began to interact on a deep level, which I normally don't do so soon after meeting someone. However, this situation was different. I asked him if he wished to speak with a pastor or minister—someone who could address his soul needs and pray with him. A short time later, I returned to his room to check on him and to do the superficial things we nurses feel we must do at such a time: give medications, check intravenous lines, and take vital signs. It was then he asked me if I would help him reach someone by telephone, and I said, "Of course."

He gave me the person's name, but the number was unlisted, so we weren't able to make the call. With his face now turned to the wall, he inquired of me, "Nurse, can I leave the hospital? There are some things I need to take care of before I go." I didn't need to ask what he meant by "go." I reassured him he was free to leave at any time, but that he would need to fill out a form that said he was doing so against medical advice. He said that was what he'd probably need to do, but he didn't leave that day.

The next day found the entire unit in an uproar. It seems my patient had been extremely uncooperative all day long, even going so far as to pull out his I.V. By the time I made my rounds and entered his room, he was dressed and ready to leave.

"What's up?" I asked in my most cheery tone, as by now, the situation was highly charged with emotion. His mother and brother were in the room with him and did not want him to leave.

"I need that form so I can sign and go," he told me, ignoring his mother's sour look. When I asked him how he'd get to his destination, he indicated his brother would take him.

The usual procedure is for the doctor to attempt to dissuade the patient from leaving the hospital, but in this case, my patient's doctor got nowhere. When I returned to his room, the doctor was handing over the form for

98

signing and writing prescriptions for him to take with him. Frail, weak, and sick, my patient was ushered into the wheelchair where he would be rolled to two or three days of freedom, at best. I felt very sad for him. As I bent to kiss his hot and gaunt cheek, he said, "I want to thank you for all you did to help me."

"If I never see you again, we'll meet in heaven," I reassured him. He nodded assent, and then was rolled away. I watched him go, and thought how proud I was of him for taking control of his life, even now, when so little seemed to be in his power. I allowed myself a brief time of tears, but then I tend to cry easily. And then I wiped my eyes and went about my business, because that is what we nurses do.

Creative Solutions

Brenda Cleary

Mrs. O. tipped the scales at 75 pounds. A petite woman of 5'2", she had end-stage emphysema, making every breath an effort. She lived at the nursing home facility where I am a certified clinical specialist in gerontological nursing (nursing of the aged).

Because of some unpleasant experiences dealing with confused patients rummaging through her personal items, Mrs. O. was very anxious about leaving such items unattended. She tried mightily to carry all of her most valuable possessions on her lap in her wheelchair, but because of her frailty, the sheer weight of the items was too much for her to carry and certainly inhibited lung expansion! So, I enlisted my husband's carpentry skills and we designed a special wooden tray for her wheelchair. With the help of the facility's activity director, Mrs. O. decorated the tray before we put the finishing touches on it and made sure it was both safe and secure.

Mrs. O. really enjoyed that tray. She was able to carry her belongings, including the ever-present Bible, with her wherever she went. Solitaire was one of her favorite pastimes, so she also used the tray to hold her cards.

I believe that having someone take a special interest in her was extremely meaningful for this unique, long-lived woman. We noticed she became more open and trusting after receiving this special gift.

Nurses can make a big difference in the lives of their patients. As our tears fell at Mrs. O's graveside service a few months ago, I observed the minimal pine box coffin which carried her to her final resting-place. I was struck by the reality that there are inequities in death as well as in life. However, I was comforted by the fact that in nursing care, even the little things can make such a huge difference in the patient's quality of life.

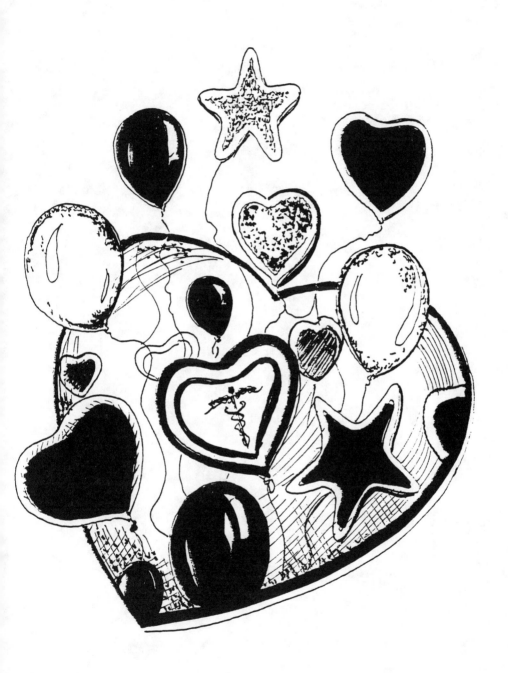

4

Humor Lightens the Load

As we move through some tense days and weeks, we need to remember that all in our lives and our workdays is not doom and gloom. Nurses like to have fun, and besides that, we know laughter is very therapeutic! Enjoy reading as we share some of the lighter aspects of the world of health care.

The Sundowner

Pamela Rogers

As a new nurse, I was ecstatic when I found out I had been hired in the neurosurgery progressive care unit at a large teaching hospital. This was somewhat of an achievement for a new graduate, since most of my fellow classmates were required to initially work on the floor in order to develop their nursing skills. The nurse manager had been impressed with my performance during my clinical rotation through the unit and felt I was ready for the challenge. Needless to say, I was overwhelmed with all the information I was expected to learn about managing the neurosurgical patient.

One evening shortly after I began my new job, I cared for an elderly patient who had fallen out of his wheelchair and sustained a bruise to the brain, which had been surgically repaired. The previous shift nurse reported to me that he sometimes had periods of confusion, mainly during the night shift. I walked into the room and greeted my patient. Perfectly pleasant and cooperative, he told me about his daughter, a physician, who had driven all the way from New Jersey to North Carolina to visit him. He spoke with pride of his daughter and her accomplishments as I listened and thought to myself, "How nice it is to have a patient who isn't confused or in a coma."

Strangely, around midnight, he became very inappropriate and agitated to the point where he required restraints to prevent him from injuring himself (and injuring me)! After a couple of hours of unsuccessful reorientation, he finally calmed down enough to sleep.

Before the first shift arrived, the neurosurgeon came in and picked up the nursing flow sheet from the bedside table. I quickly and eagerly walked over to give report.

"How did Mr. Smith do last night?" he inquired. I replied in my most professional voice, "Well, you know he was fine during the day and for the first part of my shift. He followed commands, was fully oriented, and moved all his extremities. No deficits that I could tell." The neurosurgeon listened quietly, studying the flow sheet as I continued, "But right around midnight, he became very confused and combative, and I had to restrain him." To this the neurosurgeon replied, "Oh, Sundowners." I hastened to correct him, saying, "No sir. But his daughter was down yesterday." Shaking his head and looking at me in puzzlement, the neurosurgeon turned and walked away.

The charge nurse, having overheard the conversation, called me over to the nurse's desk. Between her giggles, she informed me that "sundowners" is a term used to describe confusion that occurs at night. She explained further that it is quite common in the elderly population with this type of injury. As she spoke, I could feel the skin on my face becoming flushed and hot. I don't think I have had a more embarrassing event since in my nursing career!

The Impersonator

Julie G. Matthews

One night, as I reported to work at a local hospital, I read a memo that stated that someone had been calling the hospital and pretending to be a doctor in an effort to obtain patient information. I filed the warning away in my memory bank and began my work.

Later that night, the phone rang and I answered. A voice on the other end stated he was a certain doctor whose patients usually come to our unit. He told me he had admitted a patient and wanted to check on her condition, but could not remember her name.

He did not sound at all like himself. "What is your first name?" I asked. "I'm not telling you," he said, "I just want to know, did you get my admission tonight?" "Look," I stated, "You are sick. You really need help. Quit calling here like this and get some help for yourself. If you were really this doctor, you would tell me your first name and who your patient is." He replied, "You're not being very helpful!" I smugly hung up, knowing that I had put this creep in his place.

Later that night, the supervisor came by. I told her about the call, and her face paled as she told me about admitting one of this doctor's patients to a different unit. I froze in my tracks! What had I done?

Morning arrived. I could not face him. He came up on the floor as my shift was ending. I quickly ran to an adjoining conference room and hid behind the door. A co-worker asked, "Doc, did you call the floor tonight?" "Yes, I did," he croaked, with a voice like a frog. "Oh, by the way," he smiled, "I have laryngitis."

Hmm, Hmm Good

Lori Boisen

I took Mr. G. his morning breakfast tray a little late due to an emergency in another unit. As I put his tray down, he asked me for another glass of that wonderful apple juice, but requested that I add some ice to it this time. As I tactfully removed his Foley catheter, with the balloon intact, from his mouth, I told him I would be happy to bring him another glass of juice.

Ms. Clara's Peanut Butter Sandwiches

Jeannie Smith

I was acting as the on-call nurse for a home health agency, shuttling about from patient to patient's homes performing the standard nursing duties—catheter changes, physical assessments, etc., when I received a call to assess a patient for some cardiac and respiratory symptoms. So, I headed toward West Asheville en route to Ms. Clara's.

At the time, my Isuzu Trooper was fairly new, and I was particularly enjoying riding around in it. To tell you the truth, as I drove in the hot afternoon with my windows down and the wind in my face, I was daydreaming about how this might be like a safari. So, needless to say, I missed my turn and had to go back. I finally found the gravel driveway to Ms. Clara's green and white mobile home with a patio covered by a metal awning. Hers was the last one in the back and was shaded by a large oak tree. I pulled beside her home and reached down to get my nursing bag and straighten my nametag. As I glanced in the rear view mirror, something lying under the tree caught my eye. Taking a second look, I could hardly believe my eyes! There under the large oak tree, lined up in a single row, were about 12 freshly made, open-faced peanut butter sandwiches. Well, to tell you the truth, I have seen stranger things, so I took my nursing bag and knocked on Ms. Clara's door.

A pleasant voice invited me in and as I opened the door, I saw a pleasingly plump older lady standing in the kitchen wearing a blue cotton dress, her steel gray hair askew with small wisps falling around her face. She was happily spreading peanut butter over slices of bread. There was an open loaf of fresh bread on the counter and a jar of peanut butter nearby, with Ms. Clara adeptly smearing in swift, circular motions. As I stood there looking at Ms. Clara, she said, "Honey, would you like to help me?" This was more of a gentle command than a question, so I picked up a small metal knife and began dipping into the peanut butter. Our job was not complete until the whole loaf of bread was used and each slice placed on a large metal tray. Then Ms. Clara instructed me to take the slices outside and place them under the tree with the others.

When I came back in, Ms. Clara was sitting patiently on the couch waiting for me, and it was then that she explained how every afternoon at 4 o'clock she fed her hungry squirrels.

Ms. Clara is no longer with us, but this was one of the simple pleasures she enjoyed every day. I was privileged to have participated.

Nurse Knows Best

Jeanne M. Alford

It is difficult to be a patient, but as a nurse, it is considerably more so. I was in a terrible car accident and was literally quite broken up. I had two crushed knees that were encased in full-length leg immobilizers, and other injuries. My legs were to remain perfectly straight for eight weeks. I decided one day in my month's stay at the hospital that I would try to get myself from the chair to the bed.

How, you might ask, would such a feat be accomplished? Well, my brilliant idea was to have my nurse turn a Chux upside down on the bed and sprinkle it thoroughly with powder. I also had a foam eggcrate mattress on my hospital bed. The idea was to have me lift myself up onto the Chux and scoot myself across the bed, with my nurse and aide's assistance.

I slid all right! I slid right across the bed, met the immovable force of the eggcrate mattress, and flipped over onto my stomach and extremely painful chest, with my gown flapping in the breeze so that my considerable behind was exposed to the ceiling and to Michele and Gwen. Thank heaven I had known those two forever! What was left of my dignity? After we all realized I was O.K., we laughed very hard.

After I stopped bouncing, I just lay flat and said to Michele, "But it was such a **good** idea! I think I will just lie here for about 45 minutes, since I haven't been in any other position, except on my back, for days." I couldn't help but laugh and be exasperated at the same time. They left and returned 45 minutes later so we could all laugh some more.

The Bath

Margaret Miller

As a home health nurse in the late 70's working in a rural area, I was assigned a patient who had recently been discharged from a local hospital after having had a colostomy for cancer of the colon. The patient, Mr. S., was a retired farmer who lived with his wife in an immaculate farm house which, unfortunately, had no inside bathroom, but did have running water to the kitchen. Another challenge was that the hospital had sent him home with outdated colostomy equipment that included the old-style rubber bag and tubing. We had to make do with the supplies at hand until new supplies arrived by mail.

Since I was teaching the wife the irrigation procedure, I scheduled Mr. S. to be my first patient each day. On the second or third visit, I arrived at my usual 8:00 AM, made my assessment, changed his wound dressing, and began setting up for the irrigation. He was still quite weak, but had a great sense of humor and a very positive attitude. Our system was to set his bedside commode beside the wooden wardrobe in the bedroom and hang the irrigation bag on the door with a coat hanger.

So, on this morning, with Mr. S. sitting on the bedside commode partially clothed but draped, I hung the bag with 1000cc of tap water on the wardrobe door, ran a little water through the tubing, clamped it, and began to insert the tip of the tube into his stoma. Just then, the tubing popped off the bag and in a flash, all 1000cc of water came gushing down, covering the patient, the floor, and myself!

At first, we were all too surprised to do anything but gasp. Then, Mr. S. very calmly remarked, "Well, you said you were going to help me with an irrigation, but you didn't say anything about giving me a shower." With that, the three of us had a good laugh as I dried Mr. S. and myself and mopped up the water. It goes without saying that I was delighted to find our modern colostomy supplies had arrived when I returned the next day.

No More Cruises for Mavis!

Marcia Currier

Mavis was a frail, petite woman, barely five feet tall, with silver hair pulled back tightly and carefully braided and twisted into a bun. Her full, round face was luminous, with scarcely a line or wrinkle betraying her ninety years. Her private room was her home now, and held as many of her treasures as space would allow. The oak rocker, its finish worn with time, was rich with satiny memories of the many babies rocked to sleep in its creaking comfort. Ready to warm a sudden chill, a brightly colored granny square afghan hung across its ornately carved back.

The window box was filled with plants that Mavis had nurtured for years in her kitchen windows. Deep red geraniums with rich green leaves, delicate pink African violets, and glossy ivies filled the box. Knickknacks were scattered in among the greenery, offering the careful observer a glimpse into their caretaker's private life. Porcelain girls in hoop skirts peeked out coquettishly from ivy leaves. A china Cocker Spaniel held a leash in its mouth. Tired wicker baskets held cheerful greeting cards and precious letters from family and friends.

From the first day that Mavis came to us, I had the feeling that I knew her. After much memory searching, it came to me that she had been in charge of the hot lunch program during my high school years. The images came flooding back—Mavis in the cafeteria in her starched white uniform and beaded hair net, always impeccable. She barked orders to her co-workers and students in a manner that would make any drill sergeant proud. Always on the lookout for wastefulness, Mavis eyed each student as they passed through the line, making sure no one took more than one napkin or one straw. And woe to those unfortunate few who tried to pass off an expired lunch ticket. This would mean a quick trip to the principal's office. Mavis took no chicanery, but she did take prisoners.

Now age was beginning to cloud her once-sharp mind, and confusion crept in like a thief in the night. I'd often find her at the keyhole in the door, calling to a co-worker, possibly thinking she was at the intercom. Having spent so many years at the school, Mavis found this place in her mind to be comfortable and familiar.

I recall receiving a message from her one morning shortly after I arrived at work. Mavis never participated in any of the leisure programs, so I found it strange that she would want to see me, the activities coordinator. However, I made her room my first stop of the day. There she sat, with arms folded across her chest and a totally disgusted look on her face. Placing her unhappy demeanor aside temporarily, I said cheerfully, "Good morning, Mavis. I got your message. You wanted to see me?"

"Are you the cruise director?" she demanded.

"Well, in a manner of speaking, I guess you could say that," I replied, wondering where this was going.

"I'm very unhappy with the service I've received and I demand my money back," she hissed vigorously, shaking her finger at me. "We've been on board this ship for three days, and we've YET to leave port! I'll **never** sign up for **this** cruise again!"

Well, what could I say? I gently slipped an arm over her small shoulders, guiding her to the window. We looked out at the gentle rain; each of us lost in our own thoughts. I felt her arm slip softly around my waist.

"April showers bring May flowers," she said cheerfully, and I smiled with the knowledge that Mavis was back once again.

The Nose Knows

Barbara B. Jones

A first grade boy came into the school nurse's office very distressed. He told me he had recently undergone surgery on his nose, and was not supposed to get it hit. During recess, he was playing on the slide and hit his nose as he descended. I examined his nose closely— there were no signs of swelling, bleeding, redness, or deformities—so I questioned him about all the possible surgical procedures that could have been performed on his nose. His answer was consistently, "No." Finally, I queried, "What **did** the doctors do to your nose?" to which he replied, "They circumcised me."

Giggles from the Psychiatric Unit

Marlene Shea

Jane, a middle-aged patient, spent long hours crocheting to help her relax. Mabel's room was next to Jane's, and Mabel was confused. Often we would find Mabel standing in Jane's doorway talking with her as she crocheted. One afternoon, Jane had a pass to go home, and so was not in her room. Later that day, we found Mabel walking in the long hall with Jane's crocheting in her hands. When asked what she was doing with Jane's partially crocheted afghan, Mabel replied that she was helping Jane crochet. Unfortunately, as she "helped," she had walked the hall a number of times, unraveling about three-fourths of Jane's handwork!

Wayne was a patient who was a double amputee at the knee. Even though he had prostheses, he would often walk on his stumps. One night, a new male attendant was on duty. Unaware that Wayne was a double amputee, he made rounds with flashlight in hand and noticed Wayne's bed was empty. (Wayne had gone to the bathroom, walking on his stumps.) The attendant looked around the room, using his flashlight, when he saw two pants legs with boots hanging out from the end of the bed. As he pulled on the legs, much to his astonishment, there was no body attached!

A young licensed practical nurse came to our unit right out of training and had never been present for a code blue (cardiac arrest). One day we called a code while she was on duty. While the registered nurses were attending the code, she began moving furniture out of the room to make more space for the team to work. She opened the patient's bathroom door to put a chair in there just as the team rushed into the room, closing the nurse in the bathroom. To this day, she says her part during a code is to pray.

Back in the 70s, when I worked in a small locked unit, staff needed to call for backup from security and hospital male attendants whenever a patient was combative. One day, we had a trainee secretary on the unit, and a patient became agonistic. We told the trainee to call for help, so she picked up the phone, dialed the operator, screamed "Help" into the phone and hung up.

Junior 007 and The Young Lady in White

Helen M. Thamm

In the late 70's, an angelic-looking teenager was admitted to our mental health unit. Jamie Bondy, we'll call him, was a very polite and handsome young man. His smile melted the hearts of all the young girls and made all of us older women want to adopt him. But Jamie had one teensy, weensy, annoying little habit.

With a hairpin or paper clip, Jamie could pick any lock, or so he bragged. All his adopted moms, myself included, felt he was just kidding, until late one night around 11:00 PM. As we dragged out of the nursing office after giving report to the incoming shift, something made me look toward the polyglass door to the fire escape. There, much to my amazement, stood one of our young female schizophrenic patients. Long, wavy dark hair surrounded her pale face, and her white nightgown and robe were flowing eerily around her as she grinned with a psychotic smile. She stared off into the night sky. Looking much like an apparition from a late night thriller, she waited calmly as we raced out to rescue her before she jumped from our sixth floor wing!

But, to our surprise, we then found out she had no intention of jumping. When we reached her, she explained in her usual flat monotone, "Don't worry. He told me not to move and I would be fine!" It didn't take us long to figure out who "he" was.

Tiptoeing into Jamie's bedroom, we found the culprit lying peacefully in bed, with only a hint of a smile on his face! When I said, "All right, 007, you're busted," he couldn't refrain from laughing. Despite the fact that he had incurred strong limits due to his actions, he couldn't help gloating just a bit. After all, no one else had been able to accomplish what he had done.

He had crawled right under our noses past the nursing station, leading a psychotic girl while cleverly avoiding the security mirrors. He had picked the lock on the fire escape door, led his young charge out onto the landing, and crept back past us without anyone noticing a thing.

The next day, I suggested, in my most therapeutic manner, that he try to channel his talents in more positive and constructive ways. In my unofficial role of career counselor, I recommended to Jamie that he consider joining the CIA when he finished growing up!

A Foot Stomping Time

Petronella Arledge

Many Country and Western dancers refer to dancing as "foot stomping." Line dancers do much more stomping than boot-scooters and two-steppers, and they stomp the floor because it is part of the dance. The day I received the most severe stomping of my life, I wasn't dancing but working in surgery.

During World War II, I was a student nurse who had been in training only four short months when asked to rotate through surgery. Because of the war, training periods for various rotations were escalated due to a critical shortage of registered nurses and doctors. Military service for these two groups left huge gaps in all hospital personnel, and student nurses found themselves with responsibilities for which they weren't always totally prepared. Thus, I found myself in the surgery suite one horrendous day.

More cases were scheduled than available personnel could handle, so substitutions were made quickly. When I reported to work expecting to be a scrub nurse or a circulating nurse, I was told I'd be the doctor's assistant for a toe amputation. The shock I felt almost made me swoon, but that was nothing compared to what I was soon to feel.

Three of us made preparations in the operating room: the anesthetist, the surgeon, and me. After scrubbing, I donned my white, sterile gown and rubber gloves and carefully arranged the instruments and supplies on a table for the surgeon's use. As I helped the doctor into his surgical garb, the patient arrived on the stretcher. Immediately I noticed a pervading sickening odor. When the circulating nurse lifted the sheet from the patient's foot, my unbelieving eyes viewed toes as black as pitch in a fireplace. The surgeon explained that this patient was a diabetic who delayed treatment too long, and gangrene had set in. As we prepared to begin our unpleasant task of amputating toes, the putrid odor from the rotting flesh engulfed the three of us. Unfortunately, our masks were unable to block out all the odor. Always a person who reacted to odiferous substances, I fought my weak stomach with all the grit I could muster, but I almost lost the fight this time.

After removing the decomposing toes, the surgeon began to cauterize the remaining flesh. Just as I began to see stars and to reel from side to side, total darkness was overwhelming me. All of a sudden, I felt such excruciating pain in my feet that I was brought back to consciousness in a flash. Suddenly I realized that the surgeon was stomping my feet as if he were killing snakes! I cried out in pain as he forcefully said, "Now, let us finish our job." As I held back my tears, I regained my wits and resumed assisting.

After the surgery was over and we were out in the hall, the doctor apologized profusely. He told me, "You were about to faint on me. All I could see was white on your face and I couldn't tell where your mask stopped and your cap started. Since there was no one in the room to catch you before you hit the floor, I had to bring you back quickly, so I stomped your feet." As he spoke, my feet felt as if I would be hobbled for life. I was afraid to look at them for fear I'd see blood streaming through my shoes.

What should I have done? Bow and thank him? I did neither, but maybe I **was** a little grateful. After all, I preferred sore feet to a cracked skull.

The Payoff

Ida Chandler and Pam Tidwell

A few years ago, as part of our home health duties, Pam and I were sent out to help a confused woman who needed possible nursing home placement and a bath. Her neighbors reportedly could smell her apartment from the first floor, and she lived on the third! As we rolled her wheelchair into the bathroom, it was obvious it had been a very long time since it had been used. I washed the woman's hair in the sink, all the while thinking her hair was black or brown. As the water ran over her head, her hair turned white! Meanwhile, Pam washed the woman's body, and as she washed her back, she peeled a piece of paper off. Tossing it to the side thinking it was a piece of toilet paper, we were both surprised to see it was a $20 bill!

What Time Is It?

Jeanne M. Alford

In 1985, I cared for an alcoholic, sixty-ish, gentleman who had pancreatitis. He was on the road to recovery, but continued to need to be reoriented to place, time, and person. I went in to take care of him and reorient him for what seemed like the umpteenth time in that many days. In reorienting him, he could not tell me what day and year it was, so being the good nurse, I proceeded to tell him the year.

"It's 1885," I told him, not once but **five** times. "It's 1885." Then I walked out of his room to go down the hall. As I left his room, all of a sudden I realized what I had just done, so I quickly turned around and returned to his room to tell him about the mistake I had made. As I entered his room, I said to him, "Mr. Jones, I have something to tell you. I told you the wrong year. It is 1985, not 1885. I am so sorry for that." He looked up at me and proclaimed, "Lady, every time you come in this room I get more and more confused."

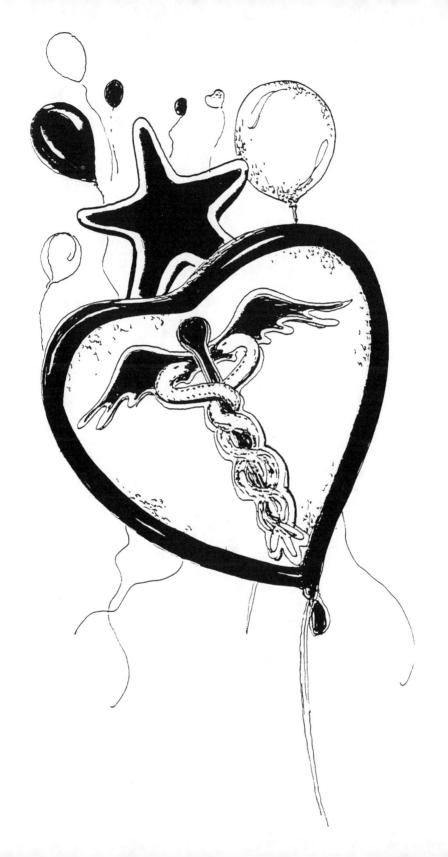

5

Medical Stretches

Nurses find ourselves in some pretty unbelievable situations from time to time. We will usually pretend nothing is wrong, and that we're not surprised by anything we see, hear, smell, or feel. This isn't always easy, however! As you read the following stories, be open to the possibility that anything is imaginable in this world and that some things simply defy explanation. But, these are some of the aspects of our job that keep it so highly stimulating from day to day. We can't be bored with unexpected happenings that occur fairly regularly! In fact, ask any nurse and you will probably get a similar response, "Nursing is just about the most stimulating profession you can join. I am rarely bored, because every day is a new day, and I'm always challenged to learn new things about people, illnesses, other health care givers, and life in general."

Our Miracle Lady

Johnna Stewart

One evening as I working in the cardiovascular lab of a 450-bed facility, we had just finished an angioplasty on a female patient, Jane, when I noticed she was extremely short of breath. She then complained of severe chest pain.

As we began to re-drape her in sterile fashion, her heart rate dropped into the 30's and her blood pressure plummeted. We quickly called a code on Jane and, even though we were performing chest compressions, she seemed awake. After approximately three unbelievable hours of CPR, during which we did everything within our power to bring Jane back to us, the code was discontinued.

Slowly, with heavy hearts, the staff left the room. I said, "Jane, please don't give up. Your daughter needs you. She can't lose another parent." (Jane's husband had passed away just three months previous). As I looked over to Jane's face, I noticed her eyes were moving back and forth. Her eyes were blinking! I quickly alerted her physician, who offhandedly said, "You're crazy. That's post-mortem movement." But then he glanced over at Jane a little more carefully, saying, "She's alive!"

She was transferred to our intensive care unit and three days later was returned to the cath lab after complaining of chest pain. Diagnostic studies showed her right coronary artery was closing again, and she was taken to emergency surgery. Again I told her not to give up and told her that I would be there to cheer her on. Five days later she was discharged.

Jane told me that she had an out-of-body experience and, touching my hand, said, "Thank you for not giving up on me." She had survived a situation that is beyond my comprehension, but one thing's for sure, she was our miracle lady!

Mr. Fuller

Cassandra Ellis

In 1993, I cared for a patient I'll never forget. I called him Mr. Fuller for reasons you shall soon see. My patient was admitted to our area with multiple diagnoses resulting in continuous oxygen and intravenous therapy, an indwelling Foley catheter, and frequent (every two hours) turning.

With the excellent nursing care he received on our unit, Mr. Fuller began to improve considerably. He soon began assisting with his own care, he fed himself without help, and his Foley was removed. Because of problems with urinary incontinence, however, Mr. Fuller continued to wear adult diapers.

After being off for four days, I returned on Saturday, and Mr. Fuller was assigned to my care. His wife told me some of the remarkable improvements in his condition, and that he was doing very well until three days ago when he stopped eating and began to complain of pain, unrelieved by medication.

Upon assessing him, I found his abdomen somewhat distended. He saturated his Attends with urine, requiring us to change them several times a day. Constipation or impaction had been ruled out as a possible cause of the distention, so we were puzzled as to what was going on.

Today, Mr. Fuller expressed to me he felt he had to urinate but could not, but I dismissed urinary retention as a possibility because of the frequent diaper changes, which were completely soaked each time. Finally, I spoke to his physician and requested an order to catheterize my patient, and was given the go ahead.

As soon as I inserted the catheter, the urine began flowing through the tube. At 800 ccs (almost a quart), I clamped the catheter for about ten minutes. At 1500 ccs, (just under a half-gallon), I clamped the catheter and emptied the bag. At 2300 ccs, I clamped the Foley once again. As my charge nurse passed by the room, I called for her to come in to see what was happening. With her as witness, I released the catheter and more urine rushed out. She left to call Mr. Fuller's physician, who came to witness this amazing event. That morning, Mr. Fuller presented us with a total of 4500 ccs of urine (over a gallon)!

After this amazing event, Mr. Fuller's abdomen was as flat as a pancake, and he was able to enjoy a nice lunch. When the next shift came on at 4:00 PM, I told them what had happened on our unit that morning, and they were incredulous. If I had not witnessed this unbelievable event, I never would have believed this was possible, but I was there for the whole thing! Believe it, it's true.

Just Another Day at School

Donna Johnson

As a school nurse, I never know what to expect from my students, but this day I got more excitement than I had ever bargained for. I usually cover three schools, and this day was my day to be at the elementary school; however, because I wanted to get my end-of-year immunization reminder letters out to over 400 sixth graders' parents, I found myself at the middle school. After working over two full days to complete the letters, I proudly carried them to the front office for mailing. As I let out a sigh of relief, I heard yelling of my name, "Mrs. Johnson! We need you! There's been a terrible accident. There's a student in the clinic with an umbrella sticking through his hand." I looked into the frightened eyes of my pale-as-a-ghost health aide who had worked in the school clinic for over 15 years and probably had more day-to-day experience in the clinic than I did.

She gasped, "I need you right now in the clinic. It's BAD." I inhaled slowly, thinking to myself, "I hope I can handle this. I hope I will know what to do." As my third year as school nurse was coming to a close, I had been teaching wellness classes in the community, performing routine screenings, and teaching CPR and first aid. Was I prepared for this? I had also worked for seven years at Busch Gardens doing first aid. Well, I thought, "Here goes. I'll give it my best."

A 12-year-old male student was out on the field playing during PE class when he happened upon an umbrella with a broken shaft. When another student tossed a ball to him thinking he would join their game, it accidentally drove the umbrella shaft right through the boy's hand. The students quickly got the coach, who "power walked" the boy to the school clinic. She sat the student down in the boys' restroom, holding his hand up with the umbrella driven through his hand.

When I arrived in the clinic, the student was sitting calmly. There was very little bleeding, so that was a relief. I instructed my health aide to call "911" and felt for the student's pulses. It was difficult to feel the radial pulse in that hand because the umbrella had exited close to the area. He sat there. He looked at me. He did not scream or cry.

As I wrapped his hand in gauze to immobilize the area as best as I could, I told him that everything would be okay. My motions were as if I was on automatic pilot. He was calm (in shock?). I felt completely numb inside, knowing that for sure I WAS in shock. Other students were very frightened. I then noticed he was getting pale, so I laid him down on a cot. His mother, who worked nearby, was on the site in five minutes, and his father arrived shortly thereafter.

Still not complaining of any pain, the student was placed in a helicopter for transport to a major trauma center. As the helicopter lifted off, we all wished him well and sighed with relief.

Luckily, the student's hand suffered no permanent damage. He recovered quickly, and was sent home to continue his recuperation. We felt grateful the injury was not serious and that a guardian angel was with this student that day. What was a freak accident turned out to be just another day at school when the day was done.

I Will Lead the Blind

Pauline Gibson

I am a Registered Nurse employed by a private physician. Acting as first assistant in surgery is one of my job duties. During June of 1996, we both realized I was having trouble focusing my eyes on the suture, and was experiencing difficulty cutting the suture. It was if my eyes were unable to focus on a certain point.

Thinking my bifocals were out of alignment, I made an appointment with my local optometrist. I realized that I had a greater problem, however, when I was asked to close my right eye and read the chart with my left. My left eye had an opaque area within its center allowing me to see around the edges, but not in the center. The optician and I were upset and his suggestion to me that I see an ophthalmologist that afternoon only served to frighten me more.

My ophthalmologist is a personal friend. He was extremely upset at his findings, and like a good nurse, I asked few questions because I sensed he did not want to be the one to give me bad news. An appointment was made for me to see a retinal specialist the next day in a nearby city.

How was I going to explain this to my family? Difficult is not an adequate word. The next day arrived, and I chose to go alone for the appointment, much to the dismay of my family and friends who wanted to be with me at this frightening time. My deep-seated faith in a higher power enabled me to continue on. My prayer was that He would be with me on this journey and that He would be my protector and helper. I was afraid my nursing career was over—I have never known of a blind nurse working in the health field. I knew that my faith had to rest in God's help because that was all there was remaining.

Sitting in my car at 6:00 AM and praying before I started out on that dark morning in June, it seemed I could feel His presence. It was dark, but I felt He was telling me He was there with me and we would make it through this day. He was the Light that would lead me.

I arrived for my appointment at 8:00 AM and learned six hours later the diagnosis for my condition: wet macular degeneration. The physician used the term legally blind to describe the vision in my left eye for the first time, and it was not pleasant. I was told that at the time, there was not an accepted medical treatment for this condition, which could have been arrested with the help of an Amsler eye chart.

The doctor informed me that one of his partners was involved in an ongoing research study of this disease and he thought I might be a candidate for the study! His partner selected patients meeting certain criteria, and with the help of a computer in Washington, DC, fifty percent were selected for a surgical procedure and fifty percent for continued medical evaluation. He emphatically stated there were no guarantees of a cure. The surgical procedure could damage my eye irreparably, and I could lose what vision I now had. After making an appointment with his partner, I made the long journey home, crying most of the way. However, I continued to feel God's presence surrounding me.

Arriving home, I found mail on my desk. In a manila envelope was one sheet of paper that slipped to the floor as I opened it. I bent to pick up the paper, which simply said, "I will lead the blind by ways they have not known, along unfamiliar paths I will guide them; I will turn the darkness into light before them and make the rough places smooth. These things will I do; I will not forsake them." (Isaiah 42:16) I knew this message was from God's mind and heart to my visual eyes. It answered all my prayer requests from the past two days. It was if God had spoken the message directly to me in my hour of need.

From where did this message come? Several weeks previous, I had written a church leader asking for information about a missions support group that I had agreed to chair. This message was from her, although there is no way she could have known about my present medical circumstances.

One bright August morning, I had the surgery that I hoped would correct the vision in my left eye. I had been chosen by the computer to undergo the operation. Now, eight months later, I have 20/30 vision in my left eye! The physician believes it was my positive attitude that allowed me to have such a remarkable recovery, but I know it was because of God's help guiding the physician's hands as he repaired my damaged eye.

My eye is not completely clear--there are a few opaque areas--but my life is in similar shape. There are still some opaque areas. I am just trying now to clean those up to make a better life for my family and me. Incidentally, I am going to Russia this year to help teach Vacation Bible School, where I will tell my story again and again.

The Christmas Miracle

Vickie Pryor

Jose was one of my favorite patients, and every morning, he was one of the first to arrive at the clinic. He had been a migrant worker, and still lived in the migrant labor camp. For the past several years, health problems had taken their toll, and he struggled with diabetes, hypertension, obesity, and leg ulcers. Unable to work harvesting vegetables, he made a meager living picking up aluminum cans along the roadways. In spite of his health problems, he always greeted me with a smile, and sometimes brought a sack of fresh vegetables for our clinic staff.

He had a large ulcer on the outside of his right ankle, and every day, I unwrapped the bandages, washed the area, applied cream, and re-bandaged the area. For the past several months, we had tried different treatments, but the ulcer just would not heal. We advised Jose to stay off his feet and keep his leg elevated, but he just smiled and shook his head. He had to keep shuffling along and picking up cans. Even though we counseled Jose about his diet, the cook at the migrant camp prepared all the meals, so Jose ate what was available.

As the Christmas holidays approached, I worried about Jose. His ulcer was growing larger, and developing a foul odor. His ankle and foot were so swollen that he could no longer wear a shoe, so he hobbled into the clinic barefooted. Christmas was on Thursday, and the clinic would be closed Wednesday afternoon through the weekend.

On Wednesday morning, as I cleansed Jose's ulcer, I showed him how to change the dressings and take care of his wound. As I explained the importance of changing the dressing every day, Jose said he'd do his best. I gathered the supplies he would need and handed them to him in a large paper bag. While I watched him slowly shuffle out the door I prayed that his ankle would improve.

The following Monday morning, Jose was waiting at the door when the clinic opened. One glance at his leg and I felt sick. "Jose, that dressing is the same one I put on your leg last week! Why didn't you change the dressing like I showed you?" Jose hung his head and replied, "I can't bend over that far, Miss Vickie. I tried, but I couldn't reach it." With a sick feeling of dread in my stomach, I unwrapped the bandages. As I began unwrapping, I asked Jose how his ankle had been feeling. "It feels pretty good, Miss Vickie. It's been itching a lot, but it doesn't hurt much," he replied.

When I removed the large gauze pad from directly over the ulcer, I was shocked to find the entire area filled with large, fat, white, wiggling maggots! They dropped off his ankle and became a wiggling mass on the linoleum floor. For several seconds, I was frozen with shock. I had never seen maggots on a patient, and I wasn't sure what to do. Finally, I grabbed a plastic basin and put it under his leg to catch the remainder of the maggots as I scraped them carefully away from the ulcer. When the site was free of maggots, I was astounded to see that the wound looked healthier than it had in months. All the tissue was pink, and it appeared to be healing well. There were no signs of infection, and the swelling was almost completely gone.

When the doctor came in to look at the ulcer, he said, "Well, Jose, that's the most unusual Christmas gift I've ever seen. The improvement in your leg is certainly a Christmas miracle. Last week, I thought your leg would have to be amputated, and now it is healing better than I ever thought possible."

In a short period of time, Jose's leg healed completely. Every year around Christmas, I think of Jose and the Christmas maggots that saved his leg.

She Wasn't Ready Yet!

Joyce Kristjansson

In the late 1970's, I cared for an 80-year-old female patient with congestive heart failure. She was very ill, and her kidneys were failing as well as her heart. In fact, her kidneys had not produced urine for over 24 hours, and the attending physician told the residents and interns to remove her Foley catheter and allow her to slip away in peace. After this discussion in the hallway, I went into her room and, much to my dismay, realized she had overheard the conversation when she opened her eyes and said to me, "I'm not ready to go yet."

I then reviewed her chart, noting that the physician had ordered the catheter to be discontinued but to keep her intravenous fluids going. I, however, did not discontinue the Foley catheter. At the end of my shift, she had a minute amount of urine in the Foley bag.

When I returned the next day, she was passing large amounts of urine. Her doctor said it was a miracle that she was still with us!

Six months later, I saw my patient once again, this time outside the halls of healing, and I realized she was my friend's grandmother.

This remarkable woman lived another 17 years, and each April, the anniversary of her amazing recovery, I received a card from her reminding me that nursing is about helping people hope until they are ready to quit hoping. In her last card to me, she wrote, "I think it is time for me to quit hoping," and two days later, she quietly and peacefully left us.

Just Lupus

Christine Blair

Alex Jones entered my life via stretcher on a July night at Lakeview Hospital, where I work as a nurse. The mechanical noise of the printer sending up admission notices broke the silence. It stated, "Alex Jones, 32, Diagnosis: Lupus, Coming from Emergency Room." Though I was working on a heart-monitored unit, this piqued my curiosity and I decided to take the admission. At least it might liven up the pace of the night.

About 10 minutes later, the Emergency Room called to give report. They described Alex as a patient chronically ill with lupus, but without any history of heart problems. His heart rate was currently in the 150 beats per minute range at rest, way too high. They felt he should be observed on a monitored unit.

In my 20+ years of nursing practice, I have cared for people of different ages, races, and diagnoses, in many situations. Formal education taught me the basics, but it's in life experience that I have learned the most. A colleague once told me that the power of natural instinct often guides medical professionals when caring for patients. It wasn't until the night I met Alex that I learned this could be true.

In my clinical knowledge, systemic lupus erythematosus (SLE) is commonly called lupus and is a disease of the musculoskeletal system. The disease, more common in women and often beginning in adolescence or early adulthood, involves chronic inflammation of the body systems. Its cause is unknown and it is usually not fatal. The most common symptom is joint pain, although inflammation can occur in any part of the body. When the ER nurse told me about Alex's heart rate in the 150s, I thought it might be due to pericarditis, which is inflammation of the lining of the heart.

When Alex arrived on the unit, he appeared much older than 32 years of age. His thinning dark hair lay matted on the pillow. He was so

133

emaciated that his dark green eyes were protruding. His appearance did not match my expectations, which were of a patient who most likely took steroids for inflammation that create weight gain and body swelling. Alex was different.

Anxious, short of breath while in bed, and wringing his hands and darting his eyes, this patient was much like a terrified child. His skin color blended into the faded cream walls of the semi-private room. Upon settling into his bed, his heart rate accelerated into the 180 range.

When I asked him his medical history to determine the cause of his current symptoms, he replied, "Just lupus." All of his medications and hospitalizations were for treatment of lupus. He denied pain, but said he was tired. After checking the orders and giving him his prescribed medication, I saw he was beginning to relax, his breathing was improving, and his heart slowed to the 110 range.

But, despite the clinical improvements, I still had a strange feeling that something just wasn't right. Remembering my colleague's advice about the use of instinct, I again asked Alex's wife about prior medical history or problems. And again they replied, "No." I added, "He looks much sicker," to which his wife replied, "He's had lupus for a long time and we have three children all under the age of five."

Still bothered by a strange feeling, I reviewed Alex's chart that included a history taken by an ER doctor and paramedics. It gave basically the same information. Since Alex's personal physician didn't work in the hospital, Alex was assigned to a group of internists.

Three hours later, about 4:00 AM, Alex's heart rate was in the over 170 and he was again short of breath and very restless. With mounting apprehension, I called the resident on call who ordered oxygen levels and a chest x-ray. Both came back normal.

"Something just doesn't look right. I just can't understand it," I said with exasperation at my inability to find any clinical data to support my feeling that something was amiss. Normal results or not, Alex's heart rate remained in the 170s, so I went to his room again to check on him. Running his words together, Alex begged, "Help me, help me, help me to breathe." The resident on call had ordered a medication for anxiety, so I advised Alex to allow the medication to take effect, reassuring him that he would feel better. I sat at his bedside until he dozed.

Two hours later, his heart monitor showed a rate of 30 and was in a very dangerous rhythm. Rushing to his room, I found him not breathing and unconscious. We called a code and emergency resuscitation efforts were begun, but Alex did not respond well. His prognosis was growing poorer, still we continued in every effort to revive Alex. The doctor who arrived first on the scene left the room to call Alex's personal physician. Fifteen minutes later, he returned to the room, announcing that while speaking to Alex's doctor, he learned that Alex needed a total heart and lung transplant, and that he had been to the finest medical centers in the area.

We worked for another hour and a half to resuscitate Alex. Now that the team had all the information about his condition, we were determined to save him. Efforts were made to move him to the top of the organ donor list, and we reserved a room in the intensive care unit for him. However, all efforts were futile, and at 7:42 AM, Alex was pronounced dead.

The team left his room in stunned silence. Neither Alex nor his family had told any medical professional in Lakeview Hospital about his desperate condition. As Alex's wife and father passed us on the way to his room, they asked, "Why?" In my heart I wanted to ask them the same question, but instead I replied with tears rolling down my cheeks, "Sometimes there isn't a reason."

In the end, I wish I would've been wrong, or knew the answer why, or that it had, after all, been "just lupus."

Contributing Author

Biographies

Biographies

Alford, Jeanne

Jeanne has worked as an intermediate critical care registered nurse at Memorial Hospital, South Bend, Indiana. Always seeking to improve patient care, she loves her patients and her profession.

Angel, Tee

Tee graduated from Florida Atlantic University College of Nursing with highest honors, where she was a member of Phi Kappa Phi Honor Society, Sigma Theta Tau International Nursing Honor Society, Iota Xi Chapter. Her writing career began in nursing school where she maintained a journal to express the phenomenology of the nursing experience.

Archeval, Ludovina

Ludovina is a staff nurse at Visiting Nurse Affiliate in Elizabeth, New Jersey. She earned a BSN and MSN from Kean University in Union, New Jersey, and plans to pursue doctoral studies while serving as adjunct professor at Kean University.

Arledge, Petronella

Petronella graduated from Hillcrest Memorial Hospital School of Nursing in Waco, Texas in October of 1946 and was a member of the United States Cadet Nurse Corps. She then spent the last 25 years of her nursing career as a school nurse, mostly at Coronado High School in Lubbock, Texas.

Blair, Christine

Christine, married four years and the mother of one son, graduated with a BSN from Eastern Michigan University in 1990. She has been writing since grade school, and is currently employed in the intermediate cardiac surgical unit at Providence Hospital in Southfield, Michigan.

Chandler, Ida

Ida, the mother of two sons and one daughter, Lives in Haw Creek, North Carolina and has worked at Visiting Health Professionals in Asheville for 18 years.

Cleary, Brenda

Brenda received a BSN and MSN from Indiana University and a PhD in Nursing from University of Texas at Austin. She is nationally certified as a gerontological clinical nurse specialist and currently holds the position of Executive Director of the North Carolina Center for Nursing.

Cooke, Tricia

Tricia is a critical care nurse with 16 years experience in a field she loves. Married for 18 years, she has two sons and is very active in Cub and Boy Scouting. She lives in North Carolina.

Dickson, Rumona

Rumona is a Lecturer, Research Synthesis at the Liverpool School of Tropical Medicine where she performs systematic reviews of the literature assessing the effectiveness of health interventions which are then disseminated to developing countries. She graduated from a hospital-based programme in Western Canada. No longer working in the area of direct patient care, she misses the joys and sorrows that came with patient contact in her clinical practice.

Ellis, Cassandra

Cassandra has worked in several areas of nursing—first as a licensed practical nurse for almost 10 years and most recently as a registered nurse. She works at Midwest City Hospital in Oklahoma City.

Flanagan, Beth

Beth received her practical nursing license in 1989 and has worked in several long-term care facilities over the years. She is currently a graduate student at Western Kentucky University pursuing a Master's degree in Humanities.

Follis, Naomi

Naomi is a graduate of Pardue University, Calumet Campus School of Nursing, with experience in intensive care and geriatric nursing. She studies with the Long Ridge Writers Group and has several articles and poems in publication.

Johnson, Donna

Donna is a school nurse in Pasco County, Florida. A native of Long Island, NY, she is a graduate of St. Vincent's Hospital School of Nursing in New York. She resides in the Tampa Bay area with husband, Don, and children, Michael and Ashley.

Lang, Lenore

Lenore is an Iowan by birth, now transplanted to South Dakota after living for 12 years in Cameroon, West Africa. She worked in orthopedics and rehab at a South Dakota hospital for 15 years and now enjoys working part-time in psychiatric nursing, which gives her the time to enjoy church and community activities.

Lederer, Ann

Ann has been a registered nurse since 1978. She is a Certified Oncology Nurse and a Certified Hospice Nurse whose article, *"Notes on a Nursing Home,"* was published in **Geratric Nursing** in 1983. Several of her poems appear in such journals as **Wind, Potato Eyes, and Pudding**.

Lewis, Carol

Carol graduated from Saint Vincent Hospital's School of Nursing in 1973 and is currently a nurse clinician in Acute Pain Service at the University of Kentucky.

Lilleby, Kathy

Kathy has served in a variety of areas of nursing—pediatrics, intensive care unit, and missionary nursing (Ecuador). She found a niche in bone marrow transplantation, first on the pediatric unit for three years then in clinical research for over 10 years. She works at the Fred Hutchinson Cancer Research Center in Seattle.

Lovell, Linda

Linda has worked in nursing since 1974, first at a local hospital then a nursing home since 1976. She feels she is serving in her right and perfect place, that her life has been enriched by each of her patients, and that it is her honor to serve God in this way.

Lynn, Ng Xiang

Ng (Lynn) lives and works in Singapore. She constantly searches for inspiration in an arid environment and hopes to write more in the future. Fatally bitten by the travel bug, she wants to see the world.

Matthews, Julie

Julie has been in nursing for over 19 years. She works in Richmond, Virginia.

Meganck, Rosemary

Rosemary is a certified nurse midwife in a full scope midwifery practice at the University of Illinois at Chicago. She received her AD in 1976, her BSN in 1990, and her MSN in 1993. She is very active in professional issues in Illinois, especially legislative issues involving Advanced Practice Nurses. Rosemary lives in a suburb of Chicago with her husband and three children.

Miller, Margaret

Margaret is presently serving as a QI/Clinical Staff Support team member for VNA of Illinois. She practiced in geriatrics for 12 years, then entered the field of public health. She has a BSN from Southern Illinois University, and a MSN from SIUE.

Nelson, Louise

Louise graduated in 1969 from the University of Connecticut School of Nursing. She has practiced in medical surgical nursing, geriatrics, oncology, home infusion, childbirth education, and telephone triage, and oncology is her first love.

Newman, Barbara

Barbara is a Senior Lecturer at The University of Sydney (Australia). Enrolled in the PhD program at the University of Technology, she has a Master of Personnel Education , numerous diplomas, and a graduate certificate in Survey Design and Data Analysis.

Poidomani, Edith

Edith is a School Nurse Supervisor in Connecticut. She holds a BS degree in Nursing from Sacred Heart University and a RN diploma from Bridgeport Hospital School of Nursing. Edith believes that the nurse, as a helping professional, needs to communicate HOPE as a way of making the difference between the quality of life and a "good" death.

Rogers, Pamela

Pamela, a staff nurse in a trauma intensive care unit at Carolinas Medical Center, was born in Germany. She holds a BS in Zoology, a Bachelors degree in Nursing, and presently attends UNCC in pursuit of a MSN in the Family Nurse Practitioner program.

Schneider, Paula

Paula has a Bachelors degree in Nursing and a Masters degree in Public Health from the University of Texas in Houston. Now residing in Florida, she is a medical writer, author, educator, and personal coach. She and her husband, Larry, own a private business, which provides in-services to people seeking practical tools for excellence in work and in life.

Schulz, Maria

Maria holds Bachelors degrees in Nursing and in Journalism. After working in the field of acute care for three years, she changed her focus to home health and has been in that sector for five years.

Shea, Marlene

Marlene graduated from St. Elizabeth Medical Center in Covington, Kentucky in 1961. Until 1974, she worked in medical-surgical nursing, and then began a career in psychiatric nursing. She presently works as Case Manager in Out-Patient Partial Hospitalization, which she helped develop in 1991. Marlene is the mother of three and grandmother of six children.

Singer, Norma

Norma lives and works in Chicago, Illinois. She is a nurse author whose stories have appeared in *Journal of the Association of Operating Room Nurses*, *Journal of Christian Nursing*, and the *Chicago Tribune Nursing News*. Additionally, she is the author of a book, *Not Old, Not Full of Days*, published in 1996 by Vista Publishing, Inc.

Smith, Jeannie

Jeannie lives in the beautiful Blue Ridge mountains in Asheville, North Carolina, where she works at Visiting Health Professionals. She has worked as a registered nurse in home health for 15 years. She lives with Tippee, Skipper, Millie (her three dogs), Callie (her cat), and her husband.

Steptoe, Terry

Terry has been a nurse for 18 years, and involved in the medical profession for 21 years. Her favorite areas have been intensive care, coronary care, and geriatrics. Married with a five-year-old son, her hobbies include horseback riding, needlework, and church activities.

Stewart, Johnna

Johnna has been in nursing since 1987 in the area of critical care. She currently works in a large cath lab, provides education to nurses, and is a writer who has been published in Who's Who in Nursing.

Taylor, Patricia

Patricia graduated from Florida State University with a Bachelors degree in Nursing in 1976 and received a Masters degree in Nursing from the University of Southern Mississippi in 1993. She is currently an associate professor of nursing at the University of West Alabama.

Tidwell, Pam

Pam currently serves as Human Resource Director at Community Care Partners. She has over 20 years of experience in home health care.

About the Editor

Paula Schneider, originally from South Texas, now lives in Tallahassee, Florida, where she is a freelance medical writer, workshop presenter, and wellness coach. With her husband, Larry, she owns a business in which she and Larry offer courses to nurses and others that are designed to reveal and nurture human potential in the workplace.

Paula holds a Bachelor's degree in nursing and a Master's degree in Public Health from the University of Texas. A registered nurse for over 22 years, she was among the First Notable Women in Texas in 1985. Throughout the years, she has discovered her niche in nursing in public health. As a public health nurse consultant and as a nursing supervisor of a local health department, Paula grew to have a deep respect for the positive role public health played in the health of the world's population. She is very interested in preventative health, health maintenance, and complementary health therapies.

Paula's mission is to "lead and inspire herself and others to personal health and wellness," and she offers wellness coaching for those who are ready to make positive lifestyle changes in order to heal.

Paula can be reached by phone at (850-877-3523. Her e-mail address is paulasch@polaris.net.

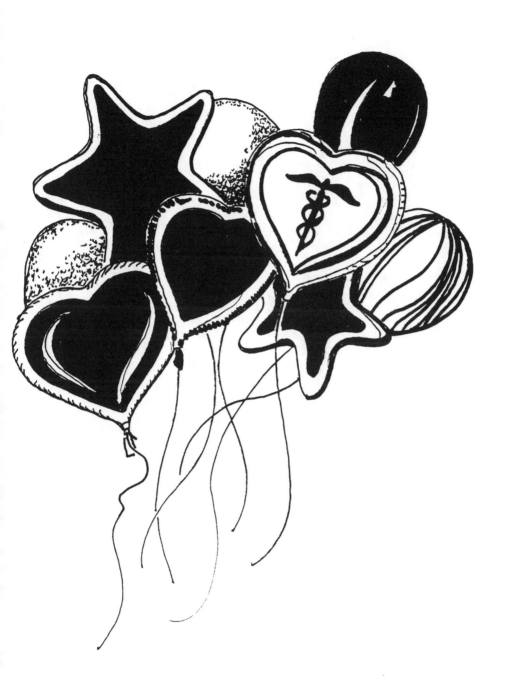